The Alkaline Diet

Reset and Rebalance Your Health Using Alkaline Foods & pH Balance Diet - Includes Top 6 Alkaline Food You Must Have in Your Daily Diet

Patricia Reed

Table of Contents

Introduction

The Alkaline Diet is a worldwide-known way to detox and fight diseases, using alkaline foods and a pH balanced diet. The diet is based on the idea that optimal health is achieved when the body's pH level is slightly alkaline. A specific diet is used to keep the body in its ideal state.

The Alkaline Diet helps you detoxify your system and get rid of accumulated acid wastes that are harmful to our health by raising the pH level of our blood (Body Ecology). This diet is for those who want to increase their energy, lose weight, and improve overall health, and prevent chronic diseases like cancer and heart disease.

It is difficult to keep an ideal pH balance because of the presence of so many chemicals, toxins and pollutants in our environment.

This Alkaline Diet tackles and offers a solution. When you follow the diet, you start feeling healthier as toxins are removed from your body, your immune system is strengthened, and improved energy levels are achieved.

The diet consists of lots of vegetables (except potatoes), fruits, grains (except rice), legumes, green tea, seeds and nuts. While meats and dairy products are eliminated from the diet, they can be eaten in moderation. Be sure that your meat is organic, or grass fed only.

You can still enjoy many of your favorite foods on the Alkaline Diet; however, be aware that you will have to be more attentive of what they are, how they affect your body and how long they stay in your system.

Why "alkaline" foods are needed

Many people have heard of the Alkaline Diet. However, most often it is accompanied by a list of foods that are alkaline such as fruits, vegetables, and grains. The main idea behind the diet is that people can eat these foods without harming themselves as well as improving their health by causing a positive change in the body. The main aim is to be able to restore an ideal body pH level which promotes health and vitality in our bodies.

So, what exactly affects our pH levels?

In order to understand how the body responds to "pH", we must understand how our bodies work at the chemical level. Our bodies are mostly made up of water, which is vital to life. Our bodies' water measures at about 65% of our total weight. The water in our body is not stagnant. Instead, it constantly flushes through the blood and lymphatic systems. carrying nutrients, oxygen and waste products.

Blood pH is the measurement of how acidic or alkaline something is on a scale of 0-14. A pH level of 7 is neutral, anything below 7 would be considered acid while anything above 7 would be considered alkaline. In the human body, pH levels are closely regulated by the presence of different chemicals which maintain homeostasis.

We maintain an ideal pH of blood and body fluids in order to maintain healthy functioning by means of buffering systems. Buffers are chemicals the body creates to help us remain at a stable state for normal functioning.

When we eat foods with either a very high or very low pH, there is an immediate reaction in our bodies to neutralize them to a more acceptable level. This is done by the kidneys. They process the foods we consume and remove excess acids or alkaline as needed. However, if these reactions are not completed, these can be stored in our tissues. When this happens, the tissue becomes inflamed, causing pain and disease.

*Homeostasis: The state of being in a constant state of equilibrium and well-being.

Repeated exposure to acidic or alkaline foods can cause an imbalance in our pH levels. This is because our bodies are made up of different types of cells with their own specific need for pH balance. For example, blood and digestive tract cells require extremely low acidity levels, while tissues such as the skin need to have a slightly alkaline condition to maintain healthy functioning.

The body does not distinguish between fat soluble and water-soluble toxins. It will process both equally through the kidneys, regardless of how toxic they are, which can lead to serious health effects over time.

It is important to maintain a balance of alkaline and acidic foods within the diet. If we consume too many acid forming foods such as meats, processed foods, sugars and grains, our bodies will be out of balance.

What foods are considered to be acid forming foods?

■ Acidic vegetables such as lettuce, radishes, spinach.

■ Sauces made with vinegar, tomato sauce and other similar products.

■ All of the fruits that are fermented, which includes vegetables as well.

■ Alcoholic beverages and non-alcoholic beverages such as soft drinks, fruit juice and tea.

Low acid fruits include:

■ All fruits excluding bananas (that contain an enzyme which can increase your body's pH level).

The goal of the Alkaline Diet is for your body to be in constant balance (homeostasis) with the food you eat. Eating too many acid forming foods has been shown to cause a great deal of damage.

Chapter 1:

What is pH?

W e all need to drink water, but not all of us know what PH is. To help eliminate any confusion, I've assembled a few quick and easy points to help those familiar with PH. PH stands for "potential of hydrogen," which gives the measure of acidity or alkalinity. It ranges from 0 to 14. The higher on this scale - meaning eight and above - the more alkaline particles are present in that solution. A perfect balance would be seven, which falls between acidic and neutral, with neither side manifesting themselves entirely at any time (although most things in nature tend to weigh more towards either acidity or alkalinity).

The higher on this scale - meaning eight and above - the more alkaline particles are present in that solution. A perfect balance would be seven, which falls between acidic and neutral, with neither side manifesting themselves entirely at any time (although most things in nature tend to weigh more towards either acidity or alkalinity). Also, It is used to test acidity or alkalinity in the body for some medical conditions.

The pH scale (sometimes referred to as the "p" scale) is a measurement of the reactivity of chemicals. A standard pH reference point is a neutral pH of 7.0, with the positive pH side, usually written as pH 7, representing more acidity. The negative side is traditionally written as pH 7 or 1, expressing more basicity. Other standard references are 5 and 10, where five represents neutral and 10 "slightly alkaline." The numbers are matched to an actual concentration of hydrogen ions [H+] in solution at that particular temperature and pressure range.

The scale is logarithmic, which means that a slight change in the PH value can cause a significant swing in its acidity or alkalinity. For example, if something has a natural pH of 4, it would take ten pH units to raise it to 5 and 100 units of pH to raise it to 6, but only 1 unit of pH to raise it from 6 to 7. That can be difficult for beginners to figure out if they're just starting with chemistry.

So why is this scale so important? Many acids, bases, and metals are dissolved in water obtained from the earth by rain. When a rainstorm hits a city or area with a large population, the water collected in those cisterns will begin to dissolve various chemicals in it. Later on, when the rain finally falls, and the cisterns empty into a stream or lake, the water may contain radioactive materials left behind by people living nearby.

This has led to an interesting question: What would happen if you took pH measurements of water in Lake Superior? As you can guess, it would be highly acidic; its pH is 7.2-7.3. So what would happen if you took some of that water and then measured its PH? It could be either strong base or strong acid, depending on where it was taken from.

So what exactly is the meaning behind this misunderstood way of measuring acids and bases? Well, it helps find out how acidic a substance is. Chemists use this scale in attempting to find out how much of something will dissolve into a liquid. The more acid a sense has, the more it can dissolve into the water to give off electrons without being absorbed by another substance.

But how did these chemicals get there? Many of them were placed on toilet seats by women who believe it will help improve their sex lives. But in reality, it does the opposite in some cases. People with solid chemical sensitivities can't stand the smell of perfumes, deodorants, or other scented items sprayed over the washroom area. This can be unfortunate because these ladies believe that spraying perfume over the seat helps them get a few "smelling" comments from other people. In reality, it's just making them sick.

Luckily, these chemicals can often be removed by simply pouring vinegar or lye (both acids) into the tank. This will cause the vinegar to break down all of the chemicals that it comes into contact with and change the water's PH. Lye is often used because it's stronger than vinegar and can be easily poured directly into a bottle and then added to the tank. Vinegar requires more dilution than lye does to break down strong scents.

PH is also used to measure how solid acids and bases are. Strong acids will have a PH of 0-2, while concrete grounds will have a pH of up to 12.

Much of this scale is based upon the symbol for hydrogen, H; the atomic weight of Hydrogen is 1.00794, meaning that it takes approximately one gram to make up 1 mole (dram) worth of hydrogen.

If you divide 2 mole's by the number itself (3.0126+3.0126), you will end up with 6.03872×10 or 60.387×10 (rounded off). This would be the square root of 6 mol of Hydrogen; therefore, it is at a pH of 7.

Now let's take a look at 7 moles: if we were to add this many moles to ourselves, we would have something that contained 49 mol of something (7×7). If you were to divide 49 by the number itself (8+8), you would end up with 6.25×10 or 62.5 (rounded off). This is the square root of 62.5 mol of hydrogen; therefore, it is at a PH of 6 (more or less).

If you were to add 8 moles to themselves, you would have 49 mol. If you divided 49 by 7+7, you would end up with 6.25×10 or 62.5 (rounded off). This is the square root of 62.5 mol of Hydrogen; therefore, it is at a pH of 6-6.2 (more or less). This is only half a decimal step away from being strictly at a physiological pH level (6-6.2).

The PH scale is like a logarithmic scale, so it is exponential.

Using the Hydrogen example, 1/10 of 1 pH unit will change the PH to 6.1-6.3 (more or less). If you went up another 1/10, then you would be at 6.4-6.5 (more or less). The scale is not linear, like the way that you might think.

Your body works at a specific level to maintain its equilibrium. Even minor changes can profoundly affect your physiology, especially if you are dehydrated and have an existing medical condition. Don't be fooled by the illusion that the body can survive on only small fluctuations in pH levels because these changes can have dramatic effects on your health (and will also contribute to premature aging).

Remember, if you change nothing else about your diet or lifestyle, avoid foods known to upset your stomach and cause acid reflux, such as coffee and alcohol. In the end, it comes down to your habits and lifestyle. If you need to avoid acidic foods, then do so. If you don't, then don't worry about it.

I am not suggesting that the average person avoid eating fruits and vegetables because they are essential for good health. I am saying that they should know how these foods can be healthily combined with others to enhance their nutritional value without causing further problems (such as excess acid).

Acidic solutions are those with a pH less than 7.0 (corresponding to a concentration of hydrogen ion [H+] above 0.01 mg/l). The body's pH must be within specific limits for the proper functioning of every cell - body cells are affected by changes in the pH level of their surroundings - and this is where many illnesses come from. The kidneys regulate the pH levels of all bodily fluids besides blood.

Our body needs a delicate balance of pH to work. A balance allows us to live and stay healthy without having to worry too much about it. Still, you must understand what this balance is and how it affects your body to avoid many diseases linked to pH imbalances.

The human body must maintain a healthy internal environment. The blood and body fluids need to maintain a certain level of acidity/alkalinity (pH) for optimal health. When the pH balance of your juices is disturbed, you can get sick. Many factors contribute to this "tipping" of our internal balance towards acidity. It all begins with the daily choices we make, such as eating habits, exercise level, type of employment, and lifestyle choices.

The most common cause for a shift in pH in our bodies is a diet high in processed foods plus sugar and sweets, stress, a lack of exercise, not enough water intake, too many toxins and pressure on the liver that lowers its capacity to neutralize acids from food and the environment.

A higher than average pH can be caused by consuming too many acid-forming foods and drinks, such as fruit juices and soft drinks, alcohol, refined carbohydrates that have been refined out of whole grains (including baking products, pasta, breakfast cereals, and sugar and white flour products), coffee, tea, colas, and alcohol.

A balanced pH in the body (within a range of 6.0 to 8.0) is required to maintain good health. Within this range, the body's tissues are preserved and healthy cells are protected from infection and toxins. No disease can take hold unless it is created in our bodies or is invading our bodies at the cellular level.

So, is there enough knowledge out there for us to make the right decisions? When we are diagnosed with an illness, it might be a case of going to the doctor and "trying" everything recommended. In reality, though, we should know that our body has its innate wisdom and unique way of handling any health problem.

Too much healthy food? Too much sleep? Too little exercise? Too little water intake? All can lead to a higher than average pH in the body. A balanced pH level in your body will help you maintain and regain your health. Healthy individuals with higher than average pH are more susceptible to various illnesses. When a pH level becomes too high, the body will find a way of correcting it - and often, we already have normal pH levels but are simply out of balance with our lifestyle choices.

Ever notice that you're more likely to get ill when the weather is damp? That's because mold thrives in humid conditions. Mold and fungi spores can easily survive in wet environments, and when these spores are floating around, they can cause a great deal of harm to your body.

It might be challenging to recognize mold allergies, but people's reactions when exposed to it are pretty severe. Some of the symptoms include fatigue, muscle pain, headache, skin irritation, and mood swings. In extreme cases, mold exposure can even lead to organ failure!

With such health risks in mind, you must take the necessary precautions to avoid any adverse effects or complications.

Chapter 2:

How Does it Affect Our Health?

Y ou can probably imagine that a slight difference in your body's pH would have profoundly adverse effects on its functioning. But just by how much? And what is the pH of an average healthy person? And why is it essential to maintain a balanced and steady state? Read on for the answers and more as we explore how pH affects our health.

To maintain a healthy body, it is essential to maintain a healthy microbial population in our gut. How does PH affect our health, and how can we keep it at an optimal level? The pH of our body reflects the balance of acidic and basic substances in the blood. It strongly influences the metabolic processes controlling acid-base equilibrium, cell growth, nutrient absorption, and muscle contraction. The average resting level for human beings is typically between 7.35-7.45 and is often referred to as acid-base equilibrium.

Our kidneys maintain this level through the excretion of acids and bases into the urine. Suppose we alter the pH level outside this range. It can have significant implications on our cells and body organs, resulting in many health issues, including increased risk of cardiovascular disease, kidney stones, and chronic fatigue syndrome.

The main factors affecting pH in our body include diet, oxygenation, exercise, and stress levels. Many foods are considered acid-forming, and others can help bring us back towards an acidic balance depending on our particular diet.

The pH of our fluid body changes depending on what's happening at the moment. Many factors influence the pH, including diet, medications, and even emotions like stress. Balancing your body naturally is one way to counteract any ill effects.

The pH scale measures acidity and alkalinity, the degree of acidity or alkalinity of a substance. A low pH on the scale can indicate rising acidity levels in the body, while a high pH indicates more alkalinity. The body's pH is measured 7.4-7.6, which is neutral. The range depends on what the body is doing at any given time—it can fluctuate upwards or downwards constantly as part of normal metabolism. It can also fluctuate when you're sick or stressed out, for example.

All life on earth is dependent upon pH levels to survive. There is a direct correlation between pH levels and the acidity or alkalinity of the body. If the pH of the blood is too acidic, this can lead to acidosis, and if it is too alkaline, this can lead to alkalosis. Each of these acidity conditions has symptoms associated with it that can be serious or even life-threatening if left untreated.

The body regulates pH levels by maintaining a ratio of hydrogen ions to bicarbonate ions within the blood. Two primary organs are involved in regulating pH in the body: The lungs and kidneys.

The lungs are responsible for the regulation of carbon dioxide and bicarbonate ions. The kidneys are responsible for maintaining calcium balance and bicarbonate ions. The kidneys also secrete hydrogen ions into the urine in ammonium ions and uric acid to maintain their proper pH balance despite external factors such as diet and stress.

If left untreated over time, alkalosis or acidosis can lead to severe health conditions, including coma or death. Acidosis can also manifest itself as hyperventilation, confusion, hallucinations, anxiety, muscle spasms, and seizures. More severe cases may include muscle spasms and unconsciousness. Alkalosis, on the other hand, may include numbness, confusion, and tingling in the extremities. More severe cases of alkalosis can lead to coma, seizures, and possibly death.

The gastrointestinal tract is another vital organ that helps regulate pH levels in the body. Many factors can affect pH levels in the gut that lead to acidity or alkalinity, including stress, diet, and medications. Some foods potentiate more acidic conditions like grains and dairy, while others increase alkaline conditions like raw vegetables and fruits.

The body also uses acid to help itself get rid of toxins. Our bodies have an endogenous killing system from the acidic environment created by the body's ability to secrete hydrochloric acid. This is nature's way of working through any sort of toxicity to bring us back into balance and health.

When the body cannot produce enough acid or makes too much acid, this can cause a whole host of problems in our digestive systems and our overall well-being. An excess amount of acidic buildup in bodily fluids can lead to life-threatening issues. When extra acidic materials are secreted from the body, they can mix with base substances and fill the bloodstream, causing severe irritation.

While there is no specific test that will diagnose acidosis or alkalosis, signs and symptoms are often associated with each of these conditions. If you have symptoms of one of these conditions, it is essential to consult with a medical professional to diagnose the situation and decide on appropriate treatment.

Bacteria also thrives on sugars found in milk when it is not pasteurized. Fermentation happens when the bacteria feed off these sugars, leading to some not-so-pleasant effects such as loose stool or diarrhea. So, it's best to drink only pasteurized milk if you want to avoid these symptoms.

Even though our body's reaction to milk might be a little unpleasant, it's essential to know how your body deals with the pH levels that milk contains. So let's get into some biology. We're going to talk about something called acidosis. It exists when the blood or other bodily fluids have a lower level of pH than expected (7.35-7.45). If we're talking about blood, this means that there is more acid than alkaline in the bloodstream, which can lead to issues such as respiratory failure and even death in extreme cases.

Acidosis can lead to several other health problems, including skeletal muscle fatigue. This is because the muscles need to be able to contract against the acidity of the blood for your body to function. If they get too much bite, they won't perform as well, which leads to a higher risk of injury.

Now that we know some of the effects of low pH on our body, let's talk about exactly how PH affects our health and why so many people are talking about it. As you can probably guess, as pH levels drop, acidity increases. When your body gets too much acidity, it's a huge sign that there will be some severe damage. It can cause bone erosion or decay, tooth erosion, and even problems with your muscles and brain.

This is why it's essential to make sure that you drink the right amount of water every day. Water helps you eliminate some of the acids that build up in your body and prevent kidney stones. The pH level that milk has been optimized for is a balance between the bacteria's acidic nature and the alkaline nature of lactic acid. This is why different kinds of milk can have other effects on your health.

When milk is not as acidic as it is supposed to, it contains a higher amount of lactose than usual. According to the International Dairy Federation, people that have trouble digesting lactose might end up with symptoms such as abdominal pain and diarrhea after drinking milk. The symptoms can usually be resolved with over-the-counter medication, but individuals need to maintain healthy body weight for bone and dental health. While you probably don't want to feel like you're going through the worst case of heartburn ever after drinking a glass of milk, the high levels of acidity in milk can be beneficial in some situations.

According to a report from Dr. Albert Schatz, acidity in food has been shown to help with nutrient absorption. This means that when you drink milk, your body can absorb calcium and vitamin D much faster. Acidity is also beneficial when it comes to digestion.

The taste of milk is fundamental in our lives. It's no secret that people will do anything to get their hands on delicious dairy products because they can do so much for our bodies. Whether you're lactose intolerant or not, it's essential to know that different types of milk have other effects on your health. By understanding the science behind all this, you can make better dietary and health decisions regarding your favorite foods.

What we found:

This study assessed the effect of acidity on the frequency and amount of gastrointestinal pathogens in milk. Researchers at Victoria University in Australia conducted it. The studies' main focus was to examine dairy farming practices as a possible cause for increased gut pathogen contamination.

The pH level of milk is essential because it aids in the growth and development of bacteria that can cause diseases like food poisoning, gastrointestinal disorders, diarrhea, vomiting, and urinary tract infections. Under certain conditions, such as disease stress, the pH level can be reduced from 7.3 to 5.5.

What we interpreted:

We found that the pH levels of milk do affect the presence and growth of gastrointestinal pathogens. This study also suggests that the bacterial population in milk is likely to result from livestock management practices rather than the chemicals used on dairy farms.

The body has a healthy balance of PH, which provides it with the proper nutrient and oxygen content in the blood. The body's PH levels can be thrown off in a variety of ways. Some of the most common methods include:

• Ingestion of excess proteins, sodium, or caffeine can lead to acidity in the body.

• Unhealthy lifestyle, such as a sedentary existence and lack of exercise. This leads to excess buildup of toxins within the body and reduces oxygen within the blood.

• Dieting or fasting causes the body to go into starvation mode, which depletes its energy resources and results in acidic conditions in the blood. This is also referred to as acidosis and can lead to severe complications over time.

• Chemotherapy and radiation treatments used to cure cancer. This causes the body to become overly acidic, which creates a variety of other serious complications.

The most common symptoms of an overly acidic body are:

• Pain in joints and muscles

• Fatigue, dizziness, and lack of energy level due to oxygen deficiency in the body. This can cause a lack of motivation and interest in daily activities.

• Excessive weight gain around the midsection, even with a healthy diet and exercise routine. An overproduction of insulin causes this due to the body's acidic environment that stores fat cells instead of burning them off as fuel for energy.

• Heart Disease and strokes have become a severe problem for a large number of people. Many of these people had no previous issues with their heart or blood vessels, leading them to believe that they are healthy. However, this can quickly result in a situation where the heart's enzymes begin to destroy its calcium reserves, leading to cardiac arrest.

• Bone deterioration occurs due to the acidic environment in the body that leads to a depletion of calcium and minerals from its stores. This can result in osteoporosis, which causes the bones to become brittle and weak.

• Generalized inflammation throughout the body starts with the digestive tract, where it begins to spread its way throughout all areas of the body. This can irritate all the organs and fatigue and mood swings that can lead to depression.

Ensure that you check your PH levels each day and address any changes that occur.

Chapter 3:

Basics of the Alkaline Diet

T he diet's premise is to manage or prevent a broad range of diseases by minimizing acidity in the blood.

What is the Alkaline Diet, and How Does it Work?

The Alkaline Diet is a way to eat that emphasizes minimizing acidity in the body. The theory behind this diet is that you can ensure healthy cell function and lower disease risk by reducing or regulating acidity in the body.

Two types of diets can be considered alkaline: vegetarian and vegan. The number one goal of an Alkaline Diet is to reduce acidity in the body by eating more alkaline-rich foods. Still, you need to be careful not to eat too many acidic foods to keep the pH balance within healthy limits.

Alkaline Diets are often recommended for people suffering from various medical conditions such as diabetes, cancer, arthritis, or gout. These diets also help people looking for weight loss solutions by stabilizing blood sugar levels and maintaining a feeling of fullness longer than with other fad diets. If you're interested in Alkaline Diets, read the following article for a detailed analysis of this diet and what foods you should eat on it.

The Alkaline Diet is a dietary style used by people who want to balance their acid-alkaline balance in the body. By eating more alkaline-rich foods, you can raise your acid levels while eating fewer acidic foods, such as most fruits and vegetables, which can increase the amount of alkalizing agents your body produces. The main goal of an Alkaline Diet is to help improve your overall health and well-being by stabilizing blood sugar levels, preventing many diseases, and promoting overall health and longevity.

The main goal of the Alkaline Diet is to balance and restore acidity in the body. When pH levels are altered, they cause pain, fatigue, mood swings, and many other symptoms. An Alkaline Diet also promotes proper digestion and boosts energy levels by increasing oxygen flow throughout the body.

In many cases, Alkaline Diets are recommended for people who suffer from various medical conditions, most commonly diabetes. When the pH levels in the body are unbalanced, the body's response is to produce more insulin to lower blood sugar levels. The problem is that it can lead to excess weight gain and high cholesterol when you have excess insulin in your blood. Many people choose to follow an Alkaline Diet because it reduces blood sugar and cholesterol levels while promoting weight loss and overall health.

Although there hasn't been enough extensive research on this topic, many people claim that an Alkaline Diet has been able to help them live a much more balanced life without feeling sleepy and tired. Many who followed the Alkaline Diet claim they wake up in the morning feeling more energized than before they started with it.

The Alkaline Diet is one of the best ways to lose weight by changing your eating habits. Since the primary goal of this diet is to reduce acidity, people who follow it often take in fewer amounts of sugar. This means that your body can't easily convert carbohydrates into fat because there's no excess sugar in your blood, to begin with. Alkaline Diets also help to prevent some diseases, which increase the risk of cancer and heart disease.

One of the most important things about an Alkaline Diet is that you need to make sure you're getting the proper vitamins and minerals. It can be challenging to achieve this when following an alkaline regimen, but it is not impossible. When you continue to follow your usual diet plan but concentrate on eating more antioxidant-rich foods, such as fruits and vegetables, you quickly feel the difference.

Although there are many reasons why people choose to go on a diet, weight loss is probably one of the main reasons why so many people are interested in the alkaline Diet. Since most of the body's processes are controlled by pH levels, having a balanced pH level is very beneficial. When you follow an Alkaline Diet for a while, you will see that you naturally begin to eat less sugar, and your body will begin to use fats more efficiently while preventing excess weight gain.

You shouldn't think that taking in too many acidic foods is good or that eating too few acidic foods is terrible – just make sure to balance all of your nutrition with whole, fresh foods so that you don't become dependent on pills or shakes.

Types of Alkaline Diets

There are several different types of Alkaline Diets that you can choose from, but not all of them are healthy for you. Many people make the mistake of thinking that a vegan diet is necessarily alkaline, but it's not even close to being one. We will now discuss the difference between vegetarian and vegan diets and show you why following either one doesn't mean that it's an Alkaline Diet.

Vegetarian Diet

A vegetarian diet is not necessarily an Alkaline Diet; it can be, but only if you eat the right foods. Vegetarians do not eat meat, and this is an important distinction. When you're on a meatless diet and don't eat any foods containing acids, such as fruits and vegetables, your body is not being fed the correct nutrients to perform at its best.

A vegetarian diet can be unhealthy because it's missing out on crucial nutrients which are essential for your body to function correctly. As described before, eating acidic foods causes the body to produce more acid to counteract the acid in the blood, leading to dehydration and excessive weight loss.

When you are a vegetarian and eat more acidic foods, you'll lose too much water and end up feeling unwell. You will also become more prone to acid reflux and acidosis because your body is not properly maintaining your blood's pH. These things can lead to many problems such as heartburn, constipation, fatigue, headaches, fatigue, and kidney stones (if you're a woman) – it all depends on what kind of lifestyle your body is accustomed to.

The only thing that vegetarians can do is add supplements explicitly designed for vegetarians, including magnesium citrate, calcium citrate, and calcium carbonate. Other than this, they will have to rely on a mixture of whole foods which are alkaline such as levitated whey protein, vegetables, fruits, and nuts.

Vegetarians can be healthy and live long lives if they take the correct supplements essential for their bodies to thrive. If you're a vegetarian reading this, I urge you to start taking these supplements to help your body succeed.

Vegans

It's very similar to an Atkins Diet but different from a vegetarian diet because they both exclude all forms of animal products such as meat and dairy products. For this reason, the vegan diet is usually high in protein and high in fat.

To keep your blood pH properly balanced, you should eat plenty of alkaline foods such as raw fruits and vegetables and cook with plenty of alkaline spices like turmeric. To maintain your balance of healthy bacteria in your gut, you need to include plenty of seeds like sesame and sunflower, and you should also ferment your foods.

Vegans need to have a good range of B12 in their diet as it's not found in any plant-based foods. There are two ways that vegans can get this vitamin, either from a supplement or a probiotic supplement, to provide them with the B12 they require. If they don't take these supplements, they could become deficient in this nutrient, and if their B12 levels drop too low, it might be fatal because the vitamin can't be stored in the body, so it needs constant intake.

One of the primary ways to do this is by limiting or avoiding foods with high levels of acidity, which include sugar, grains, processed foods, and alcohol. Foods that are more alkaline-forming in the body, on the other hand, are considered beneficial for health and include vegetables and certain fruits.

The Alkaline Diet can be summed up as a way of eating that balances acidic substances in food. The diet doesn't restrict any food items but instead focuses on balancing acids and alkaline in your body. More specifically, an Alkaline Diet includes an abundance of fruits and vegetables. When the body is maintained at a certain pH level (which is slightly more alkaline), it becomes better equipped to break down other acidic substances like alcohol, caffeine, or sugar.

It is believed that this diet works by increasing your intake of alkaline foods like fruits and vegetables, which may have the ability to neutralize your body's acidity. Some people believe that an Alkaline Diet helps improve athletic performance, especially during long runs or races. This is because an Alkaline Diet can also reduce pain and irritation in your muscles that are often associated with physical activity. In addition to this, eating more fruits and vegetables every day helps give you a natural energy boost; many people claim that they can concentrate better when eating a more Alkaline Diet.

The bottom line is that the Alkaline Diet can improve your overall well-being by protecting the body's pH balance. It is also a great idea to determine your specific pH reading, giving you a better idea of what kind of diet plan may work best for you and how best to manage it.

Is an Alkaline Diet Hard to Follow?

The good news is that an alkaline vs. acidic diet does not require you to count calories, carbs, or even measure portions. Instead, it focuses on reducing certain types of foods and increasing fresh fruits and vegetables. Fresh fruits and vegetables are a great way to eliminate unhealthy fats, control diabetes, and effectively manage your weight. If you'd like, you can try incorporating more fresh juices into your daily routine as well.

This can help you cut down on overall carbohydrate intake as well. Besides, it would help if you were avoiding processed meats as much as possible. For example, processed meats contain nitrates, which can dramatically increase acidity levels in the body and reduce overall health.

When deciding what to eat in your diet, it is essential to pay attention to your food's expiration dates. Some foods may become rancid rather quickly, and they may not even be safe for consumption after their expiration date has passed.

As you may have guessed, the key to an alkaline vs. acidic diet is to avoid certain foods like red meats and sugar. Instead, you should be reaching for fruits and vegetables that are fresh, all-natural, and organic! These foods will help you control your weight and reduce acidity levels in the body.

Chapter 4:

Starting Your Diet

W hat is the Alkaline Diet? How do I start the Alkaline Diet? What should I expect when starting the Alkaline Diet plan? These are just some of the many questions that come up when people see or hear about this new trend.

The Alkaline Diet is a dietary change in which you eat more plants, including vegetables, fruit, and nuts. Your diet should be based on whole foods; alkalizing your body is the ultimate goal of this way of eating. Some people call this a vegetarian or vegan diet because they still eat some animal foods, but they don't eat as many foods as they used to.

This way of eating is also supposed to be easier on your digestive system to get sick less often if you choose to eat this way. The diet gets more attention because it is easier on the digestive system, which is the main reason for getting sick. But this diet has many benefits, and it's not just a fad. This type of eating will help you quickly lose weight, fight disease and improve your health.

This new diet goes hand in hand with the trendy Paleo diet, which focuses more on eating hunter-gatherer foods like wild game instead of eating cornflakes and toast, but both are healthy are very good for you.

The Alkaline Diet doesn't have the same restrictions as many other Paleo-inspired diets, and there are no rules for what you can eat or can't eat. The only limitation is that you become more alkalizing in your eating, making sure to get the right amount of minerals in your system.

When most people hear about this dietary change, they think it could be difficult or challenging to pull off because of the lack of processed foods. But that isn't the case. This is a very fresh way of eating, and you don't need a lot of money or time to make it happen.

If you're not up to table scraps or wild animals, you can always get what you need from regular vegetables, fruits, beans, and nuts. You're going to want to eat more plants and fewer animal products, but you can still have eggs if that's your thing. The idea is that each person will have a different approach because we're all different, and we all have our issues with health issues that we need to address. The point is to find your version of this diet that works for you and helps you stay healthy.

If you feel like the Alkaline Diet could help you, then let's walk through what it is that you're going to want to do. In general, this is a diet where you focus on eating real food instead of processed food. You can eat fruit and vegetables as much as you want, but don't overdo it.

You can eat nuts and seeds as much as you want but go easy on the salt. If salt's a big issue for your health, then don't worry about it at all. Do what feels best for your body.

This diet is easier to pull off if you start slow and incorporate it into your regular eating habits. It would be best to take this seriously or won't see any changes in your overall health.

Please do your research on alkaline foods and learn how to eat them, where to buy them and how often to eat them. You'll want to change the way you eat for the rest of your life, so don't be afraid of learning new ways of doing things, like cooking or snacking on something healthy, when you've got a natural craving for junk food.

If you're drinking alcohol or using caffeine, you'll want to take it easy because these are not alkalinizing foods, but they don't have to be banned from your diet, either. This is a personal decision that each person has to make, and these things can be okay if they are not over-consumed by you. And if you're using table salt for some dishes, you might want to cut back on that or switch over to sea salt completely.

You might not think that the Alkaline Diet is for you or that it will fit into your lifestyle, but that's okay. You can do this diet on your own, or you can find a fitness coach or other program to help make it easy so that you don't feel guilty about it. Also, there are many different ways to go about this, so there's no need to follow everyone else's same plan.

Why Start an Alkaline Diet?

The Alkaline Diet is a lifestyle that advocates eating only certain unprocessed, alkaline-forming foods to reduce acidity in the body. Proponents believe his will prevent or treat various health conditions, including insufficient energy levels, chronic fatigue, insomnia, low immunity, and cancer. But does it work?

Do you want to lose weight quickly? Do you want to kick your acid reflux? Are you prone to kidney stones or cancer? Then maybe it's time for an Alkaline Diet. In this book, we'll cover the basics of an Alkaline Diet and why so many people are jumping on the bandwagon.

The idea is that by eating more alkaline foods, your body will release fewer acids, and therefore fewer urine salts will be converted into acids again. This creates a protective barrier around your cells, which helps them function better than they would otherwise. When your body's acid/alkaline balance is off, you can quickly pay the price. In much the same way that acidic foods can cause erosion of teeth and bones, acidity in the blood makes it harder for blood to carry oxygen, which results in tiredness. Acidic blood also makes it more difficult for cells to digest nutrients properly, weakening immunity.

Losing weight is often touted as one of the benefits of an Alkaline Diet. The claim here is that a higher Alkaline Diet encourages the breakdown of fat and limits your body's ability to store it.

Another benefit of an Alkaline Diet is that it can help those who have acid reflux, stomach ulcers, and gastritis. The theory here is that an Alkaline Diet limits the amount of acid you produce. For your body to digest food, it has to make acids to break down nutrients. For example, if you ate grains, the carbohydrates would be broken down into sugars digested into acids by the stomach.

A diet high in acidic foods can cause reflux and gastritis because it decreases the protection that your stomach's mucous membranes provide from harmful acids. The mucous membranes protect the stomach from the acids from the protein, fat, and sugar in food.

A diet high in alkaline foods may not prevent reflux, but it may slow down stomach acid production. Some people also find that they feel better after eating alkaline-rich foods, and for others, the claim of improved health seems to hold.

In some cases, the Alkaline Diet can help cancer patients because their bodies produce too much acid in response to cancer treatments or other natural stressors by creating a pro-cancer environment. These changes are believed to weaken the immune system and make your cells more vulnerable to cancer.

It may be worth considering if you find that you are having trouble losing weight or suffering from acid reflux or other gastrointestinal problems.

The Alkaline Diet is just a plant-based diet. So if you are interested in cutting out meat or eating less of it, this diet may be worth considering. The diet focuses on fresh raw foods that come from nature. The principles include limiting your meat and dairy intake, eating more vegetables, beans, grains, and nuts.

The biggest reason people are interested in the Alkaline Diet is that it can reduce the number of harmful acids entering the body when we eat food. So what's so bad about "harmful" acids? Harmful acids cause everything from arthritis, diabetes, and poor circulation to obesity, heart disease, and even cancer.

Many acids can damage cells in the body. The most often discussed ones are sulfur acids formed by eating meat, dairy, and grains. These acids form when your body breaks down food into usable nutrients.

When your body digests food, it creates several chemicals called "minerals" that it needs to operate its various systems. Some minerals dissolve into water, while others form compounds with oxygen to make them more soluble and travel through the bloodstream to other parts of your body, where they reform with iron or calcium and return to the liver for reuse.

Proponents of the diet believe that carbohydrate-rich foods are acidifying and that food should be selected from an 'alkaline' list to achieve balance. This is not about trying to lose weight. Instead, it's about eating nutrient-rich alkalizing foods intended to decrease levels of acidity.

pH stands for the potential of hydrogen. The ideal range for human blood is between 7.35 and 7.45, with an average of 7.4. The pH scale measures the potential for something to be either an acid or a base - something that donates a proton (hydrogen ion) or something that accepts a proton. If you were to compare your body's pH to that of some household substances, it would fall somewhere between battery acid and bleach.

In the body, pH levels are kept stable by a series of internal systems. One of these is the respiratory system, which takes in oxygen and exhales carbon dioxide. However, it can also be affected by several other things, including:

Diet

Health status

Tissue damage

Medications

Organic factors such as an acidic diet or high-stress levels.

Environmental factors such as strenuous exercise or exposure to pollutants and toxins

When your body digests protein, as with meat or eggs, it creates sulfuric acids that attack the soft tissues and harden them. So the minerals you get from these animal products harm your tissues while your body is using them. Your liver helps to neutralize these acids and move them out of your body through your urine. So when you eat a diet high in acid-producing foods, such as meat and dairy, you can quickly end up with more acid than you can handle each day. This leads to an acidic environment in the bloodstream, limiting oxygen flow to other parts of the body, making it difficult for those cells to operate correctly.

The first Alkaline Diet was created in the 1880s by an American dentist named George Washington Sears. He believed that acidic foods were the cause of many health problems. The basic idea is to eat food that releases tiny acid into your bloodstream. Keeping this in mind, Sears advocated for a diet high in fresh fruits and vegetables - basically, any plant-based food.

Chapter 5:

The 6 Alkaline Food You Must Have in Your Daily Diet

T he Alkaline Diet revolves around alkalizing the body to bring it back to equilibrium. And while there are many foods you can eat, you have to know what the food groups are, and which ones are beneficial to your health. But note that we all need different amounts of vitamins and minerals.

If we only eat meat or dairy, then our stomach will be acidic because the animal products don't produce much alkalinity in comparison with other foods like grains, legumes, vegetables and fruits so on this diet we should focus more on those type of foods. You can also buy liquid alkalinity in capsules to drink and take it orally.

You will be surprised that the food you are eating every day can give you a toxic environment if you are not careful and depending on what you eat, your body's acidity level will mimic that of the food. You need to know which foods are alkaline and which are acid if you really want to get healthy.

1. Vegetables and fruits:

These foods are the healthiest thing you can eat. The fiber in them helps to absorb all the nutrients in your body and its alkaline content brings your body back to a healthy pH level.

Fresh green leafy vegetables like lettuce, celery and spinach are an excellent source of chlorophyll, a marine-organically-derived alkaline substance that allows plants to photosynthesize. Chlorophyll has a high antioxidant potential that prevents oxidative damage caused by free radicals and reduces the risk of cancer.

Dark green leafy vegetables like kale, collards and mustard greens are an excellent source of vitamin K, calcium, iron and magnesium. Cruciferous vegetables like broccoli and cauliflower are also excellent sources of these minerals. They also contain a lot of fiber which is good for your digestive system.

Green cabbage is rich in potassium and has high fiber content which helps you to get rid of toxins in your body and it also has anti-cancer properties. It further prevents calcium loss from bones during the aging process. So if you want to live long this is the one for you!

Lettuce consists of 60% water which is a great source of hydrating your body and provides you with a lot of minerals and nutrients like potassium, calcium, sodium and iron.

Onions are very healthy for your body because they have an important role in stopping inflammation. They help fight bacteria and soothe arthritis pain. They can even lower the cholesterol level in your body.

Spinach is rich in vitamins, iron, calcium and fiber and it also contains polyphenols, or antioxidants that protect you from premature aging. Studies have shown that the consumption of spinach reduces the risk of cancer by up to 50%.

Avocado is one of the best things you can add to your diet because it has a lot of nutrients and minerals that are very beneficial to the health like vitamins A, E, K, C and B6, magnesium, phosphorous and potassium. It further has a high fiber content which is good for your stomach.

Vegetables may not be the only thing you need to eat if you want to get healthy. You also need to include fruits in your diet such as:

Berries are rich in fiber which makes them great for digestion. They are a source of anti-inflammatory properties due to their high phytonutrient content.

Strawberries have the highest amount of antioxidants among all fruits. These antioxidants are good for preventing oxidative stress and it also prevents inflammation and protects your body from several diseases like cancer, heart disease and Alzheimer's disease.

Grapefruit is rich in vitamin C which can help prevent cancer by reducing the growth of free radicals in your body. It has a high fiber content that provides relief from constipation and helps to control blood pressure levels by preventing water retention.

Cherries are rich in vitamin A which regulates hormone levels in your body and helps to increase your resistance to infection. It also has anti-inflammatory properties and reduces the risk of cancer.

Peaches contain high amounts of antioxidants like vitamin C which protects you against several types of cancer. They also contain a lot of fiber which helps with digestion and they help you lose weight.

Bananas are very good for your health because they contains a lot of potassium, which is very important in maintaining your heart's health, as well as fiber, Vitamin C, B6 , magnesium, iron, copper and pantothenic acid.

Figs are very good for your body because they have a high fiber content which is good for digestion. They also have a lot of potassium, calcium, magnesium, selenium and manganese.

Dried fruits such as raisins, figs and prunes are dried naturally and preserve all their nutrients which makes them an excellent snack healthy food. They help you lose weight because they have a low calorie content and they can also lower your cholesterol levels.

2. Dairy and Eggs:

Cheese can be included in your diet because it has an important role in calcium intake but only if you only eat small amounts of it because cheese is high in fat, and saturated fats aren't good for the heart. The best types of cheese to eat are feta, brie and blue cheese that have the lowest percentage of fat.

Milk is a great source of calcium because it's rich in it but you should only drink a small amount. If you want to get healthy, drink milk without any added sugar or artificial sweetener.

Eggs are an excellent source of protein and have been proven to help with weight loss by reducing your appetite. They contain high amounts of fat, so limit your consumption but make sure you don't skip breakfast since that can lead to an increase in the risk eating disorders like anorexia and bulimia.

3. Oils:

Olive oil contains only 1% fat but it is good for your heart because it has high amounts of antioxidants which help you lower your cholesterol and protect you from several diseases, and it also helps reduce the risk of cancer.

Coconut oil is one of the healthiest oils on the planet because it contains high amounts polyphenolic micronutrients which can fight inflammation, slow down the aging process in your body and kill cancer cells. It also has anti-fungal properties that help to prevent infections and wounds. this oil is used for cooking as well as in suntan lotion because it's so moisturizing.

4. Meats:

Beef is the best source of protein and has very little fat, which makes it a great source for your healthy diet. It is also very filling because it contains high amounts of aminos that help you lose weight and lower your cholesterol levels. Red meat contains no carbohydrates which makes it perfect for a diet that doesn't have carbs included.

Chicken is a great source of protein but it's not as healthy as beef because it has more saturated fat and doesn't have the same amount of fiber or omega-3 fatty acids. Chicken is a great source of vitamin B12 that helps to keep your hair and skin strong and beautiful.

Turkey/turkey breast is a perfect food for anyone just starting a healthy diet. It's not only delicious but is full of vitamins like B complex, C vitamin, and the B12 vitamin. It's lower in fat than chicken but extremely filling.

Salmon is one of the best sources of omega-3 fatty acids because they contain almost 20% of it in oily form. Omega-3s are great because they help with our cell growth, balance out our mood, heart function and fight off inflammation. Salmon is also packed with protein and is a great source of muscle building for anyone.

Mackerel is a high protein fish and great training fuel. It's a top source of omega-3 fatty acids, which are anti-inflammatory, and contains in the range of 10-11% of its calories in healthy fats. This helps to keep your body trim and healthy, giving you energy during endurance workouts or weightlifting while making you feel full with less food.

Tuna isn't just used for sushi anymore. It's a superfood containing large amounts of omega-3 fatty acids, which have been shown to fight depression and reduce inflammation. It also provides many important nutrients like protein, potassium and selenium, which are great for your health.

5. Nuts:

Nuts are one of the most powerful foods because they help you lose weight and prevent heart disease. They are also an excellent source of protein. Nuts contain healthy fats to boost your brain and keep it from aging. They also contain a lot of fiber which is good for your digestive system

Almonds can be eaten in moderation since they have high amounts of fat and calories. They're great for fighting cancer because they contain vitamin E, a strong antioxidant that protects cells from free radicals.

Pine nuts are an excellent snack because their high amounts of essential fatty acids help burn fat when consumed in moderation. They also protect from several cardiovascular diseases and help your digestive tract stay healthy.

Hazelnuts are a great source of vitamin E, magnesium and iron. They contain a lot of fiber to help you lower cholesterol levels and prevent constipation.

Walnuts are an excellent source of omega-3 fatty acids with have powerful anti-inflammatory properties that help fight off free radicals in the body. They're also high in polyphenols which are great for fighting cancer and keeping the skin young and beautiful.

6. Grains:

Quinoa is a seed which is related to spinach. It contains a lot of protein and fiber which helps you lose weight, and also contains a lot of magnesium to help your body absorb calcium better.

Brown rice helps you avoid heart attacks and strokes because it has high amounts of fiber, magnesium and manganese.

Whole grain breads help prevent cancer because they contain vitamins E, C and A that protects cells from free radicals. They're going to lower your cholesterol levels as well as protect your heart from disease or an attack. These foods will help you lose weight, fight off cancer and prevent heart disease.

Chapter 6:

Secrets to Rebalancing Your pH

Acidity levels in the bloodstream play a role in many conditions, and what's more, as we age, the body naturally makes it harder to keep our acidic levels in check. Over time, your body loses minerals and fluids needed to maintain an alkaline system in the blood.

Here are five natural ways to help rebalance your pH:

- Drink lots of water! Water is fundamental for balancing out acidity and alkalinity. Try drinking 3 liters of water per day with lemon juice squeezed into it.

- Eat lots of healthy foods high in potassium. Potassium is essential for more than just the body's blood pressure because it also helps keep our tissues alkaline.

- Eat a lot of fresh (healthy) vegetables. They are rich in potassium and minerals that can be absorbed by our bodies to alkalize them further.

- Make sure to get zinc from sources that do not include traces of lead and mercury. A zinc deficiency can cause the body to become acidic.

- Use baking soda and water to treat acidity caused by indigestion. Mix a teaspoon of baking soda in a glass of water and drink it.

This will help eliminate heartburn, nausea, bloating, and the feeling that your throat is tightening up.

I'm not sure about you, but I find it easy to become chemically imbalanced. Between the plethora of chemicals in our environment and the more natural ones in our diet, it can be tough to keep up with what is excellent and toxic. Unfortunately, living an "average" life often leaves us vulnerable to chemical imbalances that affect physical and emotional wellness.

Our pH is dynamic. When we're healthy, our bodies live within the most basic guidelines of balancing the physiochemical equilibrium and using that optimal pH as an opportunity to do good things that keep us healthy and robust. This is a pretty fantastic thing. Our bodies thrive on "perfection," or, instead, they use imperfection to survive in an environment of imbalance.

The perfection model of health has been practiced for centuries; it's why Hippocrates was so revere and his teachings are parroted by medics around the world today. The perfection model is how we are taught to think about our bodies. The hygiene hypothesis is how we think about all the chemicals that bombard us every day.

Unfortunately, this model often perpetuates the idea that a healthy body should be a chemical-free body because if we're too acidic or too alkaline, any chemical will "weaken" our body. The truth is that being too alkaline or too acidic can leave us feeling ill and like there's something odd going on inside our bodies. And so, most of us try to do something about it. We buy pH balancing pills or test strips.

But what if there was a way that you could naturally balance the pH in your body? The truth is you can! You just need to know what foods are acidic and alkaline so that you can eat them in the proper amounts.

The pH of your blood reflects the ratio of hydrogen ions (H+) to hydroxide ions (OH−) in your body. The hydrogen ion and hydroxide ion's role, or pKa, keeps harmful substances from accumulating in our bodies. When we ingest or are exposed to an acid, the pKa of the importance lowers, allowing it to be absorbed faster. On the other hand, when we consume or are exposed to an alkali like baking soda, then the pKa increases. This will allow it to be absorbed more slowly than the acid that has a lower pKa.

Deciding how much alkali or acid you should eat is hard to do on your own. For example, did you know that everything in the fruit category is sour? Or that dairy products are very high in calcium? These foods can all be good for us, but they will affect your pH balance if eaten in excess.

Calcium and Phosphorus

You might even remember it from a few years ago when the government insisted that all of us take calcium supplements to prevent osteoporosis. The truth is that calcium does not have much to do with preventing osteoporosis. It has more to do with what you eat.

Not all calcium is the same. The two primary forms are called ionic and apatite. Ionic comes from plants, while apatite comes from animals. When we've overeaten ionic or acidic calcium, we can lose bone mass because our bodies have used it for physio-chemical equilibrium and then excreted it out through our urine. This is why we lose bone mass in areas like our foreheads and hairline as we age.

The flip side of calcium is phosphorous, which our bodies need for healthy bones, energy production, digestion, and nerve function. This is why you'll find phosphorus in something like phosphoric acid, and you need it to digest your food! As with calcium, though, there are two types of phosphorous: apatite and ionic. Apatite is from animals, while ionic (phosphates) can come from both animals and plants. The problem is that too much phosphate (ionic) in the body can interfere with calcium absorption by binding to it instead of allowing it to be absorbed through our intestinal walls.

When is the pH of the blood ideal?

The ideal blood pH for us is 7.4-7.6. If we are too acidic, we can experience fatigue, pain, and low immunity. If we are too alkaline, we can experience changes in our digestive system and change in moods. The goal with nutrition and supplementation is to stay between a pH of 7 and 7.5 while maintaining an adequate intake of calcium and phosphorous to grow strong bones and maintain strong immunity against disease.

This test is cheaper than you might think, and it will help you identify which foods you should be eating more or less of. Research has shown that we are more likely to stay in an optimal pH range if we are getting between 300-600 mg of calcium and 200-400 mg of phosphorus each day.

Our bodies are pretty impressive, but that doesn't mean they can do everything on their own. We need the help of the healthy bacteria in our guts to process and utilize the food we eat to keep us healthy. If we want a better understanding of how gut health factors into our nutrition and how it plays a role in achieving strong bone density and other health goals, I would suggest checking out The Art of Healthy Guts by Rob Knight, PhD

Foods for pH balance

Fruits are alkaline foods because they contain lots of vitamin C. However, make sure you are getting enough of it and don't consume too much because excess vitamin C can increase acidity in the body. Vegetables (including leafy greens) are excellent alkaline foods. Again, make sure you are getting enough of them, and don't overdo the green veggies because they will increase the body's acidity.

Please note that fermented food is not always digested and assimilated as efficiently as "non-fermented" foods. When you eat fermented food like yogurt or kombucha, you get probiotics that will help keep your gut healthy and move it into a more alkaline state

Some supplements are designed to help us achieve this by raising our pH levels.

These supplements contain:

Magnesium malate that raises the body's pH level, maintains healthy gut bacteria, and helps with blood pressure. This supplement also helps with cell regeneration and mitochondria function. Magnesium Malate is found in many plant foods but can be found in larger quantities in green tea, bananas, grapefruit, citrus fruits, tomatoes, potatoes, watermelon, spinach greens, etc.

Methyl B12 is another supplement that raises the body's pH level and helps with metabolism and energy production. This supplement is found in smaller amounts in broccoli, cauliflower, Brussels sprouts, kale, collard greens, asparagus, liver, and other organ meats.

Glycine is a supplement that helps raise the pH level of the body and makes it more alkaline. Glycine can be found in legumes such as beans or protein powders etc.

These supplements effectively raise the pH levels in our bodies and help make us more alkaline but should not be used or overused. The goal of these supplements should be to help the body achieve an average acid/alkaline balance.

What you eat and drink

Our bodies are alkalizing or acidifying, depending on the foods we consume. While some foods have a more pronounced effect than others, we all have our favorites or "comfort foods" we like to indulge in, and that offer us some kind of emotional comfort, but as far as the body is concerned, they don't do us any favors.

A Swedish study, which was published last month in the journal Nutrition and Health, looked at the diets of nearly 30,000 men and women age 20 to 69. Compared to their peers who'd regularly consumed the most salt, subjects who ate a diet with an average of about 1,500 milligrams of sodium a day had almost twice the risk of death from any cause during six years. To put that amount into perspective, people in the study who ate about 3,000 milligrams or more each day had a 56 percent higher risk of dying over time than those who got less than 2,300 milligrams daily.

There are many natural ways to alkalize our bodies and cure what ails us. The following are some common foods, supplements, and herbs that can help maintain healthy acid/alkaline levels in the body.

Alkalizing Foods & Supplements

Cinnamon may reduce the risk of blood sugar spikes, aid digestion, and boost immune function. It also helps keep blood sugar levels low. Healthy bone formation requires a balance between acid-producing phosphorus and alkaline-producing calcium from dairy products or other calcium sources such as kale, spinach, or broccoli. The ideal ratio between calcium and phosphorous in the body is 2:1, although some people may need more calcium and others may need more phosphorous. If you find that your body is too acidic, add more alkaline foods to your diet to restore proper pH balance. Many foods can be helpful, including whole grains such as rice or wheat, beans, fruits and vegetables, nuts, seeds, and dairy products such as milk, yogurt, or cheese.

Bananas contain a natural substance called pectin that can help lower cholesterol levels. They also provide a good source of potassium, which helps regulate blood pressure and blood sugar levels.

Berries may help people with diabetes maintain stable blood sugar levels. They contain natural sugars that contribute to a fast-acting energy source for the body. You can also add these berries to your smoothies.

Unrefined salt is considered the best way to increase your body's primary mineral and trace mineral stores. Salt is also essential for digestion, ensuring that food passes through our digestive system without becoming a burden on the body's systems or being stored as waste in our organs. You can use sea salt or salted corn syrup from time to time.

Chapter 8:

Helpful Hints

An Alkaline Diet seeks to counteract excessive acidity. Fruits and vegetables naturally produce alkaline as a by-product of photosynthesis. Some people believe that eating more of these foods than acidic ones can make your body function at its best through pH balance.

The first thing you should know about an Alkaline Diet is how to calculate the pH level of foods. Acidic foods have pH values less than 7, and alkaline foods have values over 7. If you don't feel like calculating it by hand, there are plenty of apps for smartphones and tablets available for download at different app stores

There are several benefits of an Alkaline Diet, including weight loss, increased energy and stamina, better general health, and even improved athletic performance. Limit your consumption of junk food. Eating healthy does not automatically equate to eating healthy fast food. If you're used to eating unhealthy foods that don't satisfy your hunger, adjust your diet gradually by finding alternative ways to help your appetite, like by going for a walk instead of ordering a fast food meal. Take wholesome snacks with you wherever you go so that when the time comes, you're not tempted with unhealthy treats.

Pare your diet down to the foods you love and desire. Since eating healthy does not automatically equate to eating healthy fast food, enjoy everything you eat without guilt while following the Alkaline Diet. As long as you're not eating junk food 24/7 and your meals are well balanced in health-promoting foods, then you've made significant progress towards healthier eating.

Eat enough vegetables and fruits every day. Remember that you can't get all the minerals and vitamins you need from food, so taking a daily multivitamin supplement is highly recommended. Snack on produce instead of chips or potato chips for a healthier alternative. Try to eat raw veggies instead of French fries whenever possible. Salads, fruit, and yogurt are other healthy snacks on the go or between meals. Keep nuts and seeds handy as a snack if you're hungry between meals.

Avoid junk food as much as possible. Instead of eating fast food when you're hungry or between meals, try some high-fiber wholegrain bread with peanut butter or low-fat cheese to soothe your hunger pains without consuming junk food. Choose low sodium, high vitamin, and mineral enriched multivitamin. It may be expensive, but it is cheaper than the cost of an illness caused by unhealthy eating habits.

Fit regular exercise into your daily routine. Practice is good for your overall health and will help you feel more energetic and energize you for healthy eating. But remember that exercise should not be done in excess if you are trying to lose weight since research has shown that too much exercise can be counter-productive to weight control. A half-hour of vigorous activity is ideal but you can also try walking or riding your bike to work or school.

Properly prepare your food. Avoid overeating fat and ensure your meat is lean. Many popular cooking methods like deep-frying and barbecuing are destructive, so avoid preparing food the wrong way. Use all tools at your disposal to control excess fat intake, such as marinating your meat in lemon juice instead of oil.

Lower your cooking temperature to reduce any extra fats or oils that you put into a dish. The less heat you apply to a container, the less likely it is to produce off-flavors or excess lipids that can be harmful to you when eaten.

Stick with one particular type of food when you're changing your diet. Making a change in your diet can be challenging, primarily if you're used to eating different foods. Easier on the stomach and palate will be the best way to go, so stick with just fruits or organic vegetables for snacks when you're getting adjusted to the new way of eating.

If possible, learn to cook healthier foods at home instead of ordering meals from restaurants. This will save you money and encourage you to learn new methods and recipes that are healthier for you and your family.

Keep tabs on your weight. If you're not losing weight or gaining too much, you're on a healthy diet. Check yourself against current adult weight tables to see if your body mass index is slowly increasing, and make sure you are burning more calories than eating them to lose body mass.

When eating out, choose fresh foods and those less processed. The fewer ingredients used in a dish, the healthier it will be as long as you don't have any allergies or sensitivities towards any of the ingredients used.

Balance your diet. When you eat, consume the right amount of carbohydrates, proteins, and fats to provide the body with the nutrients it needs for optimal health.

For the past few decades, a diet based on alkaline principles has been popular among those interested in minimizing the risk of certain illnesses and ailments. Alkaline Diet proponents often recommend eating a variety of different plant foods and avoiding processed or refined foods.

Bear in mind that these are tips for beginners and not an ultimate list of what you need to do when following the Alkaline Diet.

· Eat more tomatoes: While tomatoes are acidic when you eat them, they work best as antioxidants once they hit your stomach. The acidity helps improve your body's ability to assimilate nutrients in other foods, which means that tomatoes will help neutralize your pH levels simultaneously.

· Drink water: One of the most common pieces of advice you will get from someone who follows the Alkaline Diet is to drink plenty of water every day. Depending on what Alkaline Diet you are tracking, you might be advised to drink more than a gallon per day or even more.

· Eat almonds: Almonds are a great source of healthy fats and energy, and because they help lower blood pressure, which is well known for being a risk factor for heart disease, they are usually listed as one of the best health foods. While almonds may help your body stay alkaline, there is no evidence showing any benefit from eating more of them.

· Use salmon oil: Some people believe that by using salmon oil, which rich in Omega-3 fatty acids, you can increase the body's ability to deal with toxins. But there isn't any evidence that consuming salmon oil will help you lose weight. It's also important to note that many of the famous fish oils on the market today have been found to contain impurities, which can cause significant health problems in some people.

· Eat more dates: Dates are a good source of simple sugars and other carbohydrates known to be healthy. They are also a good source of fiber, which helps your body feel full and fuller for longer, which means you'll probably eat less.

· Eat more spinach: The common belief is that you can help your body stay alkaline by eating more spinach, as it contains chlorophyll, vitamin K, calcium, iron, and vitamins A and C. Make sure that you are consuming a high-quality form because some spinach may contain pesticides.

· Probiotics: If you are struggling with digestive problems, it might be worthwhile to try probiotic supplements. These help to repopulate your gut with the bacteria it needs to function correctly, helping with digestion and weight loss.

Alkaline Diet Tips to Keep in Mind:

While we can't reveal every single secret about the Alkaline Diet, here are a few helpful pieces of advice to get you started on the right track when deciding to try this type of diet.

1. Following Alkaline Diet principles doesn't necessarily mean you can have a high sugar intake. Be aware that many food-based sources of sugar, including honey, fruit, and fruit juices, are high in sugar.

2. You will usually be advised to avoid processed foods, especially those with a lot of sodium. It's important to note that not all processed foods are high in sodium; canned vegetables are a good example.

3. You will be advised to eat foods containing lots of fiber, significantly as these can help fill you up while also taking longer to process through your body, enabling you to feel fuller for more extended periods. Fruit is beneficial for this purpose, but you might find it more challenging to benefit from eating refined grains.

4 . The idea behind the Alkaline Diet is that it leads you to eat more of those high antioxidants that are believed to help your body stay healthier and avoid illnesses and ailments.

5. Because Alkaline Diet advice usually tells you to be careful about how much salt you put into your food, as it can cause digestive problems, you will need to experiment a bit to see what kind of foods work best for you. This means testing different brands of spices, mixing your seasonings at home, and avoiding foods sold in packages as some may contain sodium.

6. You may be told that the best form of dairy to consume is yogurt, as this contains more beneficial bacteria than regular milk or cheese, and it's also much lower in fat and sodium. As no studies have been carried out showing that yogurt can help you lose weight, we would advise you to look for one that tastes good.

7. While the idea behind the Alkaline Diet is that you can eat as many certain foods as you like, it's probably a good idea to be careful how much fruit you consume. Although fruit can be healthy, it is also relatively high in fructose, which can cause digestive problems. If you want to lose weight, then adding less fruit than the minimum recommended amount makes sense.

8. The problem with the Alkaline Diet is that many of the foods considered healthy from this perspective aren't necessarily beneficial from a caloric or fat point of view.

9. Another problem with the Alkaline Diet is that it may only be a quick fix for weight loss. For most people, this diet won't lead to

long-term weight loss. In some cases, it might even cause weight gain as you are restricting calories to the point where your body needs energy from other sources, such as sugars and simple carbs.

10. Finally, whether you're following an alkaline or a low-fat diet, the best way to lose weight is to make sure you are eating a healthy and varied diet based on known Dietary Guidelines. This will help you eat your recommended amount of fruit and vegetables every day while ensuring that these foods contain dietary fiber, lean protein, and whole grains.

Chapter 9:
Alkaline Diet Recipes

Breakfast

Zero Grains Pancakes

Prep time: 15 minutes
Cooking time: 10 minutes
Servings: 4

Ingredients:
- ¼ cup walnuts, ground
- ½ teaspoon baking powder
- 1 teaspoon lemon juice
- 1 tablespoon Greek-style yogurt
- 1 egg white, whisked
- ½ teaspoon vanilla extract
- 1 tablespoon olive oil

Directions:
1. Mix up together the ground walnuts, baking powder, lemon juice, yogurt and whisked egg white.
2. Add vanilla extract and whisk the mixture until smooth.
3. Add olive oil and stir gently with the help of the spoon.
4. Preheat the non-sticky frying pan well.
5. Pour small amount of the smooth dough in the frying pan in the shape of the pancake.
6. Cook for 1 minute from each side over the medium heat. Serve the cooked pancakes hot!

Nutrition: calories 160, fat 13.9, fiber 0.6, carbs 4.2, protein 5

Toasts with Tofu

Prep time: 8 minutes

Cooking time: 3 minutes

Servings: 4

Ingredients:

- 4 rye bread slices
- 1 tablespoon olive oil
- ¼ teaspoon minced garlic
- ½ avocado, mashed
- 1 teaspoon cayenne pepper
- 4 oz tofu, chopped

Directions:

1. Rub bread slices with the minced garlic.
2. Preheat the frying pan and pour in olive oil.
3. Add the bread slices and cook for 1 minute on each side over the medium heat.
4. Meanwhile, mix together the cayenne pepper and mashed avocado.
5. Spread the mashed avocado mixture over the toast and add chopped tofu.
6. Enjoy!

Nutrition: calories 121, fat 9.9, fiber 2.5, carbs 6.3, protein 3.5

Overnight Fruit Oats

Prep time: 8 hours

Cooking time: 10 minutes

Servings: 4

Ingredients:

- 2 cups rolled oats

- 1 cup hemp milk

- 1 mango, peeled, chopped

Directions:

1. Put rolled oats and hemp milk in mason jars in layers.

2. Seal the lids and put the jars in the fridge overnight.

3. The next morning, add the chopped mango and stir.

4. Enjoy!

Nutrition: calories 233, fat 4.7, fiber 5.7, carbs 42, protein 7.3

Coconut Yogurt with Seeds

Prep time: 15 minutes

Servings: 4

Ingredients:

- 2 tablespoons flax seeds
- 1 oz walnuts, chopped
- 1 cup yogurt
- 1 coconut
- 1 teaspoon vanilla extract

Directions:

1. Open the coconut and remove the coconut water.
2. Discard the coconut meat and chop it.
3. Put the coconut meat, yogurt, and vanilla extract in a blender.
4. Blend the mixture until smooth.
5. Pour the cooked coconut yogurt in the glasses and sprinkle with the flax seeds and walnuts. Serve!

Nutrition: calories 460, fat 39.2, fiber 10.4, carbs 21.2, protein 9.2

Almond Millet

Prep time: 10 minutes
Cooking time: 15 minutes
Servings: 6

Ingredients:
- 2 cups millet
- 2 cups water
- 2 cups almond milk
- 1 oz almond flakes
- 1 tablespoon olive oil
- ¼ teaspoon salt
- ¼ teaspoon ground black pepper

Directions:
1. Pour olive oil in a saucepan.
2. Add millet and cook over medium heat for 1 minute.
3. Add salt and ground black pepper and stir.
4. Add water and almond milk. Stir well and close the lid.
5. Cook the millet for 15 minutes over medium heat or until the millet soaks up all the liquid.
6. When the millet is cooked, stir it and transfer to serving bowls.
7. Sprinkle with the almond flakes and serve!

Nutrition: calories 485, fat 26.7, fiber 8, carbs 53.5, protein 10.2

Morning Kale Salad

Prep time: 15 minutes

Cooking time: 10 minutes

Servings: 4

Ingredients:

- 14 oz kale
- 4 oz sunflower seeds
- 3 tablespoons almonds, chopped
- 1 teaspoon paprika
- ¼ teaspoon minced garlic
- ½ teaspoon pink salt
- 1 tablespoon agave syrup

Directions:

1. Chop the kale roughly and place in the salad bowl.
2. Blend together the sunflower seeds, almonds, paprika, minced garlic, and pink salt.
3. Add agave syrup and blend mixture until smooth.
4. Pour dressing over the chopped kale and stir.
5. Let the salad rest for 10 minutes.
6. Then stir it one more time and serve!

Nutrition: calories 258, fat 16.9, fiber 4.7, carbs 21.6, protein 9.9

Fennel Salad

Prep time: 10 minutes

Servings: 4

Ingredients:

- 1 cup radishes
- 12 oz fennel bulb
- 4 oz jicama
- ½ lime, juice
- 3 tablespoons avocado oil
- ¾ teaspoon salt
- 1 tablespoon almonds, chopped

Directions:

1. Slice the radishes, fennel, and jicama and place in large bowl.
2. Sprinkle the salad mixture with the lime juice, avocado oil, and salt.
3. Stir gently and sprinkle with the chopped almonds.
4. Enjoy!

Nutrition: calories 67, fat 2.3, fiber 5.4, carbs 11.5, protein 2

Oat Patties

Prep time: 10 minutes

Cooking time: 5 minutes

Servings: 2

Ingredients:

- 1 cup rolled oats
- ¼ teaspoon salt
- 1 egg white
- 2 tablespoons almond milk
- 1 tablespoon olive oil
- 1 tablespoon flax seeds

Directions:

1. Grind the rolled oats and mix together with the salt, almond milk, and flax seeds.
2. Whisk the egg white and add it to the rolled oat mixture.
3. Stir the mixture well until a smooth and homogenous texture.
4. Make medium patties from the rolled oat mixture.
5. Cover a baking tray with parchment and place the patties on it.
6. Cook the patties for 5 minutes at 365 F.
7. Then let the cooked patties chill and serve!

Nutrition: calories 277, fat 14.4, fiber 5.4, carbs 29.7, protein 8.2

Mint Smoothie

Prep time: 15 minutes

Cooking time: 5 hours

Servings: 2

Ingredients:

- 4 oz almonds, raw
- 5 dates, pitted
- 1 ½ cup almond milk
- 2 oz mint leaves
- 2 teaspoons chia seeds
- ½ cup ice
- 1 tablespoon cocoa powder

Directions:

1. Chop the dates and place them in the food processor.
2. Add raw almonds and almond milk.
3. Add mint leaves and chia seeds.
4. Add cocoa powder and ice.
5. Process the mixture until smooth at maximum speed.
6. Pour the smoothie into glasses and enjoy!

Nutrition: calories 444, fat 38.1, fiber 10.2, carbs 23.8, protein 10.2

Fro-Yo

Prep time: 10 minutes

Servings: 2

Ingredients:

- 1 banana, chopped, frozen
- ½ cup almond milk
- ½ tablespoon coconut nectar
- 1/3 teaspoon almond butter
- 1 tablespoon chia seeds
- ¼ teaspoon ground cinnamon

Directions:

1. Blend together chopped the banana and almond milk until smooth.
2. Add coconut nectar and almond butter.
3. Then blend the mixture for 1 minute more.
4. Add chia seeds and stir.
5. Pour the cooked Fro-Yo in the glass and serve!

Nutrition: calories 244, fat 18.3., fiber 5.8, carbs 20.9, protein 3.8

Main Dishes

Fragrant Avocado Gazpacho

Prep time: 10 minutes

Servings: 4

Ingredients:

- 1 cup tomatoes, chopped
- ¼ cup water
- 1 chili pepper, chopped
- 1 teaspoon chili flakes
- ½ teaspoon salt
- 1 tablespoon lemon juice
- 2 avocados, chopped
- 2 cucumbers, chopped
- 1 teaspoon minced garlic
- 1 teaspoon white pepper
- ½ cup fresh parsley, chopped

Directions:

1. Place tomatoes, chili pepper, avocado, cucumber, and parsley in a blender.
2. Add water, chili flakes, salt, lemon juice, and white pepper.
3. Blend mixture until smooth.
4. Pour the cooked gazpacho into the glasses and serve immediately!

Nutrition: calories 242, fat 20, fiber 8.5, carbs 17.1, protein 3.7

Alkaline Pilaf

Prep time: 15 minutes
Cooking time: 25 minutes
Servings: 2

Ingredients:
- ½ cup quinoa
- 1 white onion, diced
- 1 cup water
- ½ teaspoon salt
- ¾ teaspoon nutmeg
- ½ teaspoon paprika
- ½ teaspoon ground black pepper
- ½ cup fresh cilantro, chopped
- 1 oz spinach, chopped
- 1 tablespoon coconut oil

Directions:
1. Preheat oven to 365 F.
2. Place the coconut oil in the baking tray and melt it.
3. Add the diced onion and quinoa.
4. Stir mixture well.
5. Add water, salt, nutmeg, paprika, ground black pepper, cilantro, and spinach.
6. Stir pilaf mixture and cover with foil.
7. Place the pilaf in the oven and cook for 25 minutes or until all liquid is absorbed. Serve and enjoy!

Nutrition: calories 249, fat 9.9, fiber 5.1, carbs 34.1, protein 7.3

Parsnip Puree

Prep time: 10 minutes

Cooking time: 25 minutes

Servings:3

Ingredients:

- 10 oz parsnip, peeled, chopped
- 1 tablespoon coconut oil
- 1 teaspoon salt
- ½ teaspoon ground turmeric
- 1 cup water
- 1 carrot, chopped

Directions:

1. Preheat oven to 365 F.
2. Put coconut oil on the baking tray.
3. Add chopped parsnip and carrot.
4. Add water and sprinkle the vegetables with the ground turmeric and salt.
5. Place the baking tray in the oven and cook for 25 minutes or until all vegetables are soft.
6. Then transfer the vegetable mixture in the blender or use a potato masher to make the puree.
7. Serve warm.

Nutrition: calories 120, fat 4.9, fiber 5.2, carbs 19.2, protein 1.3

Hot Asparagus

Prep time: 25 minutes
Cooking time: 3 hours
Servings: 2

Ingredients:
- 14 oz asparagus
- 1 tablespoon coconut oil
- 1 teaspoon chili flakes
- ½ chili, chopped
- 1 tablespoon Greek yogurt
- 1 teaspoon salt
- ½ lemon
- 1 tablespoon olive oil
- 1 teaspoon flax seeds

Directions:
1. Chop asparagus roughly and sprinkle with chili flakes, chili, and salt.
2. Squeeze lemon over asparagus and stir the vegetables. Leave for 10 minutes to marinate.
3. Place coconut oil on the baking tray and melt it.
4. Preheat oven to 365 F.
5. Place the asparagus on the baking tray and sprinkle with the flax seeds.
6. Add Greek yogurt.
7. Cover the baking tray with the foil and transfer in the oven.
8. Cook the asparagus for 20 minutes. Enjoy!

Nutrition: calories 229, fat 15.6, fiber 4.9, carbs 12.8, protein 13.4

Sweet Potato Halves

Prep time: 15 minutes

Cooking time: 2 hours

Servings:2

Ingredients:

- 2 sweet potatoes, halved
- 1 teaspoons coconut oil
- 1 teaspoon salt
- ½ teaspoon turmeric
- ½ teaspoon chili flakes

Directions:

1. Mix up together salt, turmeric, and chili flakes.
2. Then add the coconut oil and blend mixture.
3. Rub potato halves with the coconut oil mixture and wrap in the foil.
4. Place the potatoes in a preheated oven to 365 F and cook for 15 minutes or until soft.
5. Chill the sweet potatoes land serve!

Nutrition: calories 23, fat 2.3, fiber 0.2, carbs 0.7, protein 0.1

Tender Onions

Prep time: 15 minutes

Cooking time: 20 minutes

Servings: 4

Ingredients:

- 4 white onions, peeled
- 1 oz cilantro, chopped
- ½ teaspoon salt
- 1 teaspoon dried parsley
- 4 teaspoon olive oil
- 1 teaspoon flax seeds
- 4 teaspoons Greek style yogurt
- 1 cup water

Directions:

1. Make holes in the onions and sprinkle holes with the salt, dried parsley, olive oil, flax seeds, and yogurt.
2. Pour water in saucepan and place onions.
3. Close the lid and simmer onions for 30 minutes over the low medium heat or bake in the oven at 365 F for 20 minutes.
4. Serve warm!

Nutrition: calories 111, fat 6.7, fiber 2.7, carbs 11.6, protein 2.2

Cauliflower Salad

Prep time: 15 minutes

Cooking time: 10 minutes

Servings: 2

Ingredients:

- 10 oz cauliflower, chopped
- 1 oz pomegranate seeds
- 2 tablespoons olive oil
- ½ teaspoon turmeric
- 3 tablespoons lemon juice
- 1 teaspoon fresh mint
- 1 oz fresh parsley, chopped
- 2 tablespoons Greek yogurt

Directions:

1. Sprinkle chopped cauliflower with olive oil and turmeric.
2. Place the cauliflower in the oven and bake for 10 minutes at 365 F.
3. Combine chopped parsley, fresh mint, and lemon juice and stir.
4. Put cooked cauliflower in a bowl and add pomegranate seeds.
5. Add parsley mixture and stir salad well. Enjoy!

Nutrition: calories 179, fat 14.5, fiber 4.4, carbs 11.8, protein 3.7

Sweet Potato with Filling

Prep time: 15 minutes
Cooking time: 1 hour
Servings: 2

Ingredients:
- 2 sweet potatoes
- 2 oz black beans, cooked
- 1 oz red onion, chopped
- 1 cup fresh spinach, chopped
- 1 avocado, chopped
- 2 tablespoons lime juice
- 3 tablespoons olive oil
- ½ teaspoon minced garlic
- ½ teaspoon salt

Directions:
1. Make long cuts in the sweet potatoes and put in oven.
2. Bake the sweet potatoes for 40 minutes at 400 F or until soft.
3. Meanwhile, mash the avocado and mix it with the chopped spinach, chopped onion, lime juice, olive oil, minced garlic, and salt. Stir mixture well.
4. Add black beans and stir. When sweet potatoes are cooked, remove from oven and scoop half the sweet potato meat.
5. Fill the sweet potatoes with the avocado mixture. Enjoy!

Nutrition: calories 504, fat 41.1, fiber 11.9, carbs 32.4, protein 8.9

Lentil Pilaf

Prep time: 10 minutes
Cooking time: 23 minutes
Servings: 6

Ingredients:
- 8 oz asparagus, chopped
- 1 teaspoon salt
- 1 tablespoon olive oil
- 1 cup lentils, cooked
- ½ cup water
- 1 garlic clove, chopped
- 1 onion, chopped
- ½ teaspoon ground black pepper
- 1 tablespoon lemon juice
- 1 tablespoon sesame oil

Directions:
1. Place the chopped asparagus in a saucepan and add olive oil. Sauté the asparagus for 3 minutes.
2. Then add salt, chopped garlic, and onion.
3. Add ground black pepper and lemon juice.
4. Sprinkle the mixture with the sesame oil and ground black pepper. Stir mixture well and add water.
5. Close lid and sauté for 10 minutes over medium heat. Add the cooked lentils and stir the pilaf until homogenous.
6. Close the lid and cook the pilaf for 10 minutes more. Let the cooked pilaf chill little and serve!

Nutrition: calories 170, fat 5, fiber 11, carbs 22.8, protein 9.4

Marinated Beets

Prep time: 20 minutes
Cooking time: 30 minutes
Servings: 2

Ingredients:
- 11 oz beet, peeled, sliced
- 2 tablespoon olive oil
- 1 teaspoon minced garlic
- ½ cup water
- ½ teaspoon salt
- 1 teaspoon chili pepper
- 3 tablespoon lemon juice
- 1 teaspoon cumin

Directions:
1. Preheat the oven to 365 F. Place the beets on the baking tray and sprinkle with the water.
2. Cover the beets with the foil and bake for 30 minutes or until tender.
3. Meanwhile, mix up together the olive oil, minced garlic, salt, chili pepper, lemon juice, and cumin. Stir well.
4. When the beets are cooked, chill well.
5. Brush with the garlic mixture and leave for 10 minutes to marinate. Enjoy!

Nutrition: calories 201, fat 14.7, fiber 3.5, carbs 17.2, protein 3.1

Side Dishes

Stuffed Avocados

Prep time: 15 minutes

Servings: 2

Ingredients:

- 1 tomato, chopped
- ¼ cup spinach, chopped
- ½ cucumber, chopped
- ½ red onion, chopped
- ½ teaspoon ground black pepper
- ¼ teaspoon minced garlic
- 1 tablespoon olive oil
- 1 avocado, pitted, halved

Directions:

1. Mix up together the chopped tomato, spinach, cucumber, and red onion.
2. Sprinkle the vegetables with the ground black pepper, minced garlic, and olive oil. Stir the vegetables carefully.
3. Fill the avocado halves with the vegetable mixture. Enjoy!

Nutrition: calories 296, fat 26.8, fiber 8.3, carbs 15.8, protein 3.2

Garlic Eggplant

Prep time: 20 minutes

Cooking time: 7 minutes

Servings: 4

Ingredients:

- 2 eggplants
- 1 teaspoon salt
- ½ teaspoon ground black pepper
- 1 teaspoon minced garlic
- 2 tablespoons olive oil

Directions:

1. Slice eggplants lengthwise. Sprinkle the eggplants with the salt and leave for 10 minutes.
2. Mix up together ground black pepper, minced garlic, and olive oil.
3. Rub eggplants with the garlic mixture well.
4. Preheat the grill skillet.
5. Place the eggplants in grill skillet and cook for 1 minute from each side. Enjoy the meal immediately!

Nutrition: calories 130, fat 7.5, fiber 9.8, carbs 16.5, protein 2.8

Sauteed Mushrooms

Prep time: 10 minutes

Cooking time: 20 minutes

Servings: 4

Ingredients:

- 12 oz mushrooms
- 1 yellow onion, sliced
- 2 tablespoons coconut oil
- ½ teaspoon smoked paprika
- ½ teaspoon cayenne pepper
- ¼ cup fresh parsley, chopped

Directions:

1. Place coconut oil in the skillet and melt.
2. Slice the mushrooms. Place the mushrooms in the skillet and cook for 3 minutes. Stir the mushrooms from time to time.
3. Then add sliced onion.
4. Sprinkle vegetables with the cayenne pepper and smoked paprika.
5. Stir mixture and close the lid. Sauté the vegetables over the low heat for 15 minutes. Stir the cooked meal and serve!

Nutrition: calories 91, fat 7.2, fiber 1.7, carbs 5.9, protein 3.2

Healthy Potato Salad

Prep time: 10 minutes
Cooking time: 10 minutes
Servings: 6

Ingredients:
- 1 cup red potatoes, halved
- ½ cup broccoli, chopped
- 1 sweet pepper, chopped
- 1 onion, chopped
- 1 cucumber, cubed
- 2 tablespoons olive oil
- 1 teaspoon salt
- ½ teaspoon turmeric

Directions:
1. Steam red potatoes and broccoli until the vegetables are soft.
2. Meanwhile, place the sweet pepper and cucumber in a large bowl.
3. Sprinkle the vegetables with the salt and turmeric.
4. Add onion and stir well.
5. When the vegetables are cooked (potatoes and broccoli), place them in the bowl.
6. Sprinkle the salad with olive oil and stir. Enjoy!

Nutrition: calories 82, fat 4.9, fiber 1.6, carbs 9.6, protein 1.4

Grilled Zucchini

Prep time: 15 minutes

Cooking time: 4 minutes

Servings: 4

Ingredients:

- 1 zucchini, sliced
- 1 teaspoon minced garlic
- 2 tablespoons olive oil
- ½ teaspoon ground nutmeg
- 1 teaspoon salt
- 1 teaspoon chili flakes

Directions:

1. Sprinkle the sliced zucchini with the minced garlic, olive oil, ground nutmeg, salt, and chili flakes.
2. Stir well and leave for 5 minutes.
3. Meanwhile, preheat the grill.
4. Thread the zucchini into the skewers and transfer to the grill.
5. Cook the zucchini for 4 minutes totally.
6. Serve hot!

Nutrition: calories 70, fat 7.2, fiber 0.6, carbs 2, protein 0.7

Indian Vegetables

Prep time: 15 minutes
Cooking time: 15 minutes
Servings: 2

Ingredients:
- ½ teaspoon fresh ginger, grated
- 1 chili pepper, chopped
- 1 teaspoon minced garlic
- ½ onion, sliced
- 10 oz cauliflower, chopped
- 1 tomato, diced
- 2 tablespoons olive oil
- 1 teaspoon curry powder
- 1 teaspoon mint
- ½ teaspoon salt

Directions:
1. Preheat the pan well. Add olive oil.
2. Add chopped chili peppers, cauliflower, onion, and tomato. Stir well.
3. Sprinkle vegetables with the curry powder, mint, and salt.
4. Add ginger and remaining ingredients.
5. Stir the vegetables and roast for 5 minutes.
6. Meanwhile, preheat the oven to 365 F.
7. Place the roasted vegetables in the oven and cook for 10 minutes more.
8. Chill the cooked vegetables and serve!

Nutrition: calories 180, fat 14.4, fiber 5.1, carbs 12.9, protein 3.7

Marinated Cucumbers

Prep time: 15 minutes

Cooking time: 10 minutes

Servings: 1

Ingredients:

- 1 cucumber
- ½ teaspoon lemon zest
- 2 tablespoons lime juice
- ¼ teaspoon salt
- 1 teaspoon cayenne pepper
- 2 tablespoons olive oil
- 1 oz fresh cilantro, chopped

Directions:

1. Chop cucumber into medium pieces.
2. Mix together the lemon zest, lime juice, salt, cayenne pepper, olive oil, and fresh cilantro.
3. Stir mixture well.
4. Combine the chopped cucumber and oil mixture. Stir well and leave for 15 minutes to marinate.
5. Enjoy!

Nutrition: calories 309, fat 28.8, fiber 3.1, carbs 16.9, protein 3

Grilled Peppers

Prep time: 5 minutes

Cooking time: 5 minutes

Servings: 2

Ingredients:

- 2 sweet peppers
- 1 teaspoon minced garlic
- 1 tablespoon olive oil

Directions:

1. Grill the sweet peppers from each side for 2 minutes.
2. Then cut the grilled sweet peppers into the strips. Remove the seeds.
3. Sprinkle the pepper strips with the minced garlic and olive oil. Stir the meal.
4. Enjoy!

Nutrition: calories 100, fat 7.3, fiber 1.6, carbs 9.5, protein 1.3

Olive Salad

Prep time: 10 minutes

Servings: 4

Ingredients:

- ¼ cup green olives, pitted
- 1 cup cherry tomatoes
- 1 cup lettuce
- 1 tablespoon olive oil
- ½ teaspoon salt
- ½ cup fresh parsley, chopped

Directions:

1. Slice the olives and chop the lettuce roughly.
2. Transfer the vegetables to a bowl.
3. Cut the cherry tomatoes into halves.
4. Add tomatoes to the bowl.
5. Add parsley and sprinkle salad with olive oil and salt.
6. Stir the salad gently and serve!

Nutrition: calories 43, fat 3.7, fiber 0.9, carbs 2.7, protein 0.7

Apple Salad

Prep time: 15 minutes

Servings: 2

Ingredients:

- 1 sour apple
- 1 carrot, peeled
- 1 tablespoon pomegranate seeds
- 1 tablespoon lemon juice
- ½ teaspoon olive oil
- ¼ teaspoon ground cinnamon

Directions:

1. Cut the apple and carrot into strips and place them in a bowl.

2. Add pomegranate seeds and lemon juice.

3. Then add olive oil and ground cinnamon.

4. Stir the salad gently and serve immediately!

Nutrition: calories 96, fat 1.4, fiber 3.8, carbs 21.8, protein 0.7

Snacks and Appetizers

Protein Balls

Prep time: 10 minutes

Servings: 4

Ingredients:

- 2 oz almonds, crushed
- 3 oz pumpkin seeds
- 3 tablespoons almond butter
- 1 tablespoon chia seeds
- ½ teaspoon agave syrup

Directions:

1. Place almonds, pumpkin seeds, and chia seeds in a blender.
2. Blend mixture well.
3. Add the almond butter and agave syrup and blend mixture for 30 seconds more.
4. Make the small balls from the almond mixture and serve !
5.

Nutrition: calories 282, fat 24.1, fiber 4.4, carbs 10.5, protein 11.1

Sweet Potato Chips

Prep time: 7 minutes

Cooking time: 20 minutes

Servings: 6

Ingredients:

- 3 sweet potatoes, peeled
- 1 teaspoon olive oil
- 1 teaspoon cayenne pepper

Directions:

1. Slice sweet potatoes and sprinkle with the olive oil and cayenne pepper.
2. Place the sliced sweet potatoes on a baking tray.
3. Preheat the oven to 365 F.
4. Transfer the tray to the oven and cook for 20 minutes or until the sweet potatoes turn into the chips. Serve!

Nutrition: calories 8, fat 0.8, fiber 0.1, carbs 0.3, protein 0.1

Avocado Fries

Prep time: 15 minutes

Cooking time: 17 minutes

Servings: 6

Ingredients:

- 1 avocado, pitted, peeled
- 2 tablespoons sesame seeds
- 2 tablespoons olive oil
- 1 pinch salt

Directions:

1. Cut avocado into fries shape.
2. Blend together sesame seeds and olive oil.
3. Add salt and stir well.
4. Coat the avocado fries with sesame seed mixture.
5. Preheat oven to 325 F.
6. Put avocado fries on a baking tray
7. Cook the avocado fries for 17 minutes in the oven.
8. Chill the avocado fries and serve!

Nutrition: calories 126, fat 12.7, fiber 2.6, carbs 3.6, protein 1.2

Delicious Balls

Prep time: 15 minutes

Servings: 7

Ingredients:

- 3 tablespoons rolled oats
- 2 tablespoons rice protein powder
- 1 tablespoon almond butter
- 1 teaspoon flax seeds
- ¼ teaspoon ground cinnamon
- ¼ teaspoon vanilla extract
- 1 tablespoon agave syrup

Directions:

1. Put the rolled oats, rice protein powder, flax seeds, and ground cinnamon in a bowl.
2. Add agave syrup, vanilla extract, and almond butter.
3. Mix with a spoon until homogenous.
4. Make the small balls of the cooked mixture and enjoy!

Nutrition: calories 44, fat 1.5, fiber 0.9, carbs 4.9, protein 3

Nori Snack

Prep time: 15 minutes

Cooking time: 2.5 hours

Servings: 8

Ingredients:

- 4 nori sheets
- 2 tablespoons sesame oil

Directions:

1. Preheat the oven to 260 F.
2. Cut the nori sheets into the quarters and brush with sesame oil. Place the nori sheets on a baking tray and transfer to the oven.
3. Cook the snack for 10 minutes. Enjoy!

Nutrition: calories 35, fat 3.4, fiber 0.5, carbs 0, protein 0.5

Crispy Garbanzo Beans

Prep time: 5 minutes

Cooking time: 20 minutes

Servings: 6

Ingredients:

- 1 cup garbanzo beans, cooked

- 2 teaspoons coconut oil

- 1 teaspoon cayenne pepper

- ½ teaspoon ground black pepper

Directions:

1. Mix the garbanzo beans, coconut oil, cayenne pepper, and ground black pepper.
2. Stir mixture and place on baking tray.
3. Preheat oven to 370 F.
4. Transfer the baking tray to the oven and cook for 20 minutes or until crispy.
5. Chill the cooked snack and serve!

Nutrition: calories 136, fat 3.6, fiber 5.9, carbs 20.5, protein 6.5

Delicious Soynuts

Prep time: 10 minutes

Cooking time: 15 minutes

Servings: 5

Ingredients:

- 6 oz soybeans
- 1 teaspoon salt
- 1 tablespoon olive oil

Directions:

1. Mix soybeans, salt, and olive oil.
2. Preheat the oven to 365 F.
3. Place the soybeans on a baking tray and transfer to the oven.
4. Cook the soybeans for 15 minutes. Stir from time to time.
5. Enjoy!

Nutrition: calories 176, fat 9.6, fiber 3.2, carbs 10.3, protein 12.4

Tomato Salad

Prep time: 8 minutes

Servings: 4

Ingredients:

- 1 cup cherry tomatoes
- ½ cup fresh cilantro, chopped
- 1 garlic clove, chopped
- 1 tablespoon olive oil

Directions:

1. Cut cherry tomatoes into halves and place in large bowl.
2. Add chopped cilantro, garlic clove, and olive oil.
3. Stir well and enjoy!

Nutrition: calories 40, fat 30.6, fiber 0.6, carbs 2.1, protein 0.5

Baked Tofu

Prep time: 8 minutes

Cooking time: 16 minutes

Servings: 2

Ingredients:

- 8 oz firm tofu
- 1 teaspoon olive oil
- 1 teaspoon mint
- ¼ teaspoon ground black pepper

Directions:

1. Cut tofu into cubes and sprinkle with the olive oil, mint, and ground black pepper.
2. Preheat the oven to 360 F.
3. Place the tofu on a baking tray and put in oven.
4. Cook the tofu for 16 minutes. Stir from time to time.
5. Chill the cooked tofu to room temperature and serve!

Nutrition: calories 100, fat 7.1, fiber 1.2, carbs 2.2, protein 9.4

Desserts

Aromatic Figs

Prep time: 8 minutes

Cooking time: 3 minutes

Servings: 4

Ingredients:

- 4 fresh figs
- 1 teaspoon agave syrup
- ¼ teaspoon ground cinnamon
- ¼ teaspoon ground cloves

Directions:

1. Make cross cuts in the figs and sprinkle them with agave syrup, ground cinnamon, and ground cloves.
2. Preheat the oven to 400 F.
3. Place the figs in the preheated oven and cook for 3 minutes.
4. Serve the cooked figs immediately!

Nutrition: calories 53, fat 0.2, fiber 2, carbs 13.7, protein 0.7

Purple Mash

Prep time: 10 minutes

Servings: 2

Ingredients:

- ½ cup almonds
- 1 cup blueberries
- 3 tablespoons coconut flakes
- 2 bananas
- ¾ cup almond milk
- ½ teaspoon vanilla extract

Directions:

1. Place the almonds and blueberries in a blender and blend well.
2. Then peel the bananas and add to blender. Add almond milk and vanilla extract.
3. Blend the mixture until smooth.
4. Place the purple mixture in the bowls and add coconut flakes. Stir well and enjoy!

Nutrition: calories 521, fat 36.5, fiber 10.5, carbs 48.8, protein 9.2

Banana Fritters

Prep time: 10 minutes

Cooking time: 7 minutes

Servings: 6

Ingredients:

- 4 bananas, peeled
- 1 tablespoon lemon juice
- 3 tablespoons coconut flakes
- 1 tablespoon almond butter
- 1 teaspoon ground cinnamon

Directions:

1. Mash the bananas with a fork and combine with the lemon juice, coconut flakes, and ground cinnamon. Stir it until homogenous.
2. Place the almond butter in a skillet and melt it.
3. Make medium fritters from the banana mixture with a spoon and place in hot almond butter.
4. Cook the fritters for 30 seconds on each side.
5. Serve the cooked fritters hot!

Nutrition: calories 97, fat 2.6, fiber 2.8, carbs 19.2, protein 1.6

Orange Ice Cream

Prep time: 10 minutes

Cooking time: 3 hours

Servings: 4

Ingredients:

- 1 cup Greek style yogurt

- 1 orange

- 1 teaspoon liquid Stevia

- ½ teaspoon ground cinnamon

- ½ teaspoon vanilla extract

Directions:

1. Cut the orange into the halves and juice tit with the help of the juicer.
2. Then whisk together the yogurt and orange juice. Add ground cinnamon and vanilla extract. Stir well.
3. Place the yogurt mixture in the ice cream molds and transfer to the freezer. Freeze mixture for 3 hours.
4. Serve and enjoy!

Nutrition: calories 174, fat 11.6, fiber 1.3, carbs 11.7, protein 4.9

Sweet Pumpkin

Prep time: 10 minutes

Cooking time: 10 minutes

Servings: 4

Ingredients:

- 12 oz pumpkin, peeled
- 1/3 cup agave syrup
- ½ teaspoon ground cinnamon
- ½ teaspoon ground ginger
- 1 teaspoon coconut oil

Directions:

1. Cut the pumpkin into the medium cubes and place in the saucepan.
2. Add agave syrup and sprinkle with the ground cinnamon, ground ginger, and coconut oil.
3. Stir well and leave for 10 minutes.
4. Simmer the pumpkin for 15 minutes over medium heat. Chill the cooked dessert and serve!

Nutrition: calories 124, fat 1.4, fiber 2.7, carbs 29.4, protein 1

Sweet Cashew Cream

Prep time: 5 minutes

Cooking time: 10 minutes

Servings: 4

Ingredients:

- 1 cup almond milk

- 2 oz cashews

- 1 teaspoon vanilla extract

- 1 tablespoon coconut flakes

- 1 tablespoon agave syrup

Directions:

1. Blend almond milk, cashews, vanilla extract, and agave syrup.

2. When the mixture is smooth, add coconut flakes and pulse for 3 seconds more.

3. Transfer cooked cream to a bowl and let it chill in the fridge for 10 minutes. Serve and enjoy!

Nutrition: calories 243, fat 21.3, fiber 1.9, carbs 12.5, protein 3.6

Fig Paste

Prep time: 10 minutes

Servings: 4

Ingredients:

- 2 mangos, chopped
- 1 banana, chopped
- 5 figs, chopped
- 2 cups orange juice
- 1 teaspoon ground cinnamon

Directions:

1. Put mangos and banana in a blender.
2. Add figs and blend mixture until smooth.
3. Add orange juice and ground cinnamon. Blend the mixture for 30 seconds more.
4. Transfer the paste into bowls and serve immediately!

Nutrition: calories 244, fat 1.2, fiber 6.4, carbs 60.5, protein 3.4

Raw Banana Cake

Prep time: 15 minutes

Cooking time: 20 minutes

Servings: 6

Ingredients:

- 6 tablespoons rolled oats
- 4 bananas
- ½ cup strawberries
- ¼ cup almond milk
- 1 teaspoon vanilla extract
- ¼ cup agave syrup
- 1 tablespoon almond butter

Directions:

1. Blend together the bananas, strawberries, almond milk, and almond butter.
2. Add agave syrup and vanilla extract. Blend until smooth.
3. Mix the rolled oats and banana mixture. Stir until blended.
4. Place the mixture in the pie mold and press well.
5. Let the pie rest for 20 minutes and cut it into pieces. Enjoy!

Nutrition: calories 177, fat 4.5, fiber 3.3, carbs 4.5, protein 2.4

Almond Balls

Prep time: 11 minutes

Cooking time: 10 minutes

Servings: 4

Ingredients:

- 3 oz figs
- 4 dates
- 1 tablespoon sesame seeds
- 1 oz almonds, chopped
- 1 tablespoon almond butter
- ¼ teaspoon vanilla extract

Directions:

1. Blend figs, dates, and almonds until smooth.
2. Transfer mixture to a bowl and add almond butter and vanilla extract.
3. Stir it well until blended.
4. Make small balls with a teaspoon and place in the freezer.
5. Freeze the balls for 10 minutes and enjoy!

Nutrition: calories 156, fat 7.2, fiber 4.3, carbs 22.6, protein 3.7

Chapter 10:

Supplements That Increase pH Balance

F or those new to the pH conversation, pH levels can determine whether you're acidic or alkaline. It's essential to have balance for the body to feel good and function optimally. We will now provide some of the most common supplements that doctors around the world widely recommend.

We all know that pH balance is essential for a healthy body, but did you know it's also necessary to maintain optimum oral health? By balancing your pH throughout the day, you can prevent illness and discomfort. When all is said and done, we're only human. It's impossible to live without polluting the environment with some sort of toxin — these small things are a part of life.

As long as they help you feel better, get rid of excess weight, or give energy, why not indulge your taste buds every once in a while? And if you're looking for the right supplements that increase pH balance, this is the book for you. pH test strips are easy to use, and you can check your pH in the comfort of your own home. Learn more about how to increase pH balance.

Your body's pH balance, also known as the acid-alkaline balance, varies with time and activity. This is the process of neutralizing excess acid in your body by converting it to alkali — an agent that becomes highly concentrated in blood plasma (hemoglobin) and creates a buffer effect on the entire system. While it's essential to maintain a healthy and balanced pH level of 7.2, any outside factors that can influence the balance are dangerous.

Some of the most effective supplements that increase pH balance that you can start using right away!

1. Olive oil: This versatile buttery oil contains monounsaturated fatty acids that are easy on the stomach.

2. Chocolate: What better way to aid in oral health than by eating some of the world's most delicious desserts? Remember to stick with dark or semi-sweet chocolates when picking out a piece of chocolate. Milk or white chocolates contain extra sugar that can increase your risk for tooth decay and other oral diseases.

3. Pomegranate: This juicy fruit has been used for centuries to treat gum disease and bad breath. The pomegranate is an excellent source of vitamin C, which is essential for keeping gums strong. Eat it fresh, dried, or in juice.

4. Pineapple: It's hard to believe that some people avoid pineapple because of its high sugar content. Although this tropical fruit is a bit high in calories, you can easily control your intake by sprinkling it on top of yogurt or salsa, blending it into smoothies, or eating the fresh pieces with a mouth full of toothpicks.

5. Wheatgrass juice: This powdery green vegetable is packed with vitamins and minerals, so it's a great way to supplement your diet.

6. Psyllium husk: This joint fiber supplement is easy to add to food, but it also has rich health benefits. Psyllium husk comes from the seeds of the Plantago plant and can help relieve many gastrointestinal issues while keeping your mouth healthy and your bowels regular.

7. Spirulina: This tiny blue-green alga is a nutritional powerhouse that fights off harmful bacteria. You only need to consume ½ teaspoon daily for its immune-boosting properties. Add it to yogurt, smoothies, or juice for a nutritious treat!

8. Apple cider vinegar: One of the most discussed topics in regards to pH levels is the apple cider vinegar diet. Apple cider vinegar helps increase the pH levels by making the body more alkaline. Many people have talked about how this is a great way to detox your body and help you lose weight at the same time. It's also recommended for those who suffer from high blood pressure and even acid reflux or heartburn. This is one reason why so many people swear by apple cider vinegar on Pinterest to cure these problems.

9. Baking soda: You can use baking soda as part of your baking recipes and sprinkle it on your food, but most people do not do that. Instead, you'll find that people are using it in their coffee, as a bubbling bath, or even to wash their hair.

Consider that baking soda is not a highly concentrated form of pH balancing agents and isn't the same as baking powder. It doesn't work exactly like that, and to use it properly, you'll want to combine it with vinegar. Baking soda is negatively charged, while vinegar is positive. When combined, they neutralize each other's effects on the body. This means that they balance each other out and give you the best possible results.

10. Cinnamon: Many people have tried different types of cinnamon to help with weight loss or cure various infections. If you have any kind of bacterial infection, then it's suggested that you take cinnamon supplements. As far as weight loss goes, cinnamon isn't going to give you dramatic results, but it will help. Many people take it because they believe that it will help them kick-start their metabolism and burn fat faster. While this isn't the case, taking cinnamon can help with the frequency of your bowel movements and how quickly they are carried out. This is important because this ensures that your body has enough energy and removes toxins effectively enough for the body to function well.

11. Garlic: Garlic has antibacterial properties that can improve your body's immune system and overall health, but it also has a considerable impact on pH balance. Taking garlic supplements will increase your pH levels and make you more alkaline. There are many different pills or capsules that you can take to achieve this effect, but it is suggested you go with the medications because they are easier to use and won't harm your stomach. Take these capsules at least four times a day for optimum results.

12. Epsom salt baths and foot soaks: Epsom salt is used to balance the minerals in your body, primarily magnesium and calcium, both necessary for bone health. When you soak in Epsom salt baths, you get a small dose of alkalinity, which is thought to help your body absorb magnesium. When you wash your feet in Epsom salt, the magnesium stays in your system longer and can aid in blood clotting and healing.

13. Dietary magnesium: Lacking dietary magnesium can lead to poor absorption of calcium because it treats it as a toxin. Still, through pH balancing, the body releases the calcium stored inside tissues and begins to use it for bone formation. If you are not getting enough dietary magnesium, the body will continue to hold on to the calcium for much longer.

14. Orange juice: If you have an acidic body, you need to drink at least five glasses of fresh orange juice per day. Orange juice provides a boost for antioxidants and vitamin C, which dramatically affects your immune system. There are several other benefits, but one thing you can count on is that this combination will help neutralize the excess acid in your body so it won't become an issue in the future.

15. Vegetables: A healthy and Alkaline Diet consists of lots of fresh vegetables. This includes leafy greens, broccoli, cabbage, and any other type of vegetable you can get your hands on. Vegetables have a very high concentration of antioxidants which neutralize the acids in your body. By introducing fresh vegetables into your

diet, you'll also notice increased energy levels and faster recovery after physical activity.

16. Water: Most experts agree that we should consume at least 2 liters of water per day to keep our body clean and free from acid in the blood. This is because some foods we eat have a powerful effect on the pH level in our bodily fluids. Water is the best alkaline agent you can get, and it's readily available, so there's no reason why you shouldn't have it available 24/7 to keep your body clean and functioning correctly.

17. Tomatoes: Tomatoes contain loads of antioxidants and other alkalizing nutrients like vitamin C. They're very effective at neutralizing acidic substances in your body, like uric acid, produced by the breakdown of purines. If your diet contains too much protein, tomatoes will balance things out naturally.

Beans: Beans are another highly alkalizing food you can add to your diet to increase your body's bodily fluids' pH levels. Beans provide fiber that helps remove toxins from the digestive tract, and there's also a decent amount of antioxidants as well so eating beans is a great way to boost overall health.

Many other supplements can help achieve a healthy pH balance and ensure that every part of your body is as healthy as possible, including the skin, hair, and nails. Different types of diets and drinks will make the most of this process. This is where taking control of yourself and knowing what's best for you is crucial.

Acidic bodily pH can cause any number of health problems. Fortunately, some supplements can help balance your pH at home.

1) Dietary changes: Talk to a doctor or health professional about the types of foods you should be eating more and which you should limit. Foods high in protein, fiber, vitamins, and minerals will provide better hydration and an alkaline environment for the body.

2) Alkaline supplements: There are various supplements on the market made specifically to promote a higher level of alkaline in your body. Most are taken in pill form, but the ingredients are primarily found in most fruits and vegetables.

3) Detoxifying your body: Be sure to drink plenty of water throughout the day to flush out body toxins. Exercise regularly and avoid caffeine or alcohol daily since they can slow or stop the detoxification process.

4) Water pH test: Use a home water pH test to determine how acidic or alkaline the water you're drinking is. If it's near 7, it's neutral; however, most tap water comes in at 5-6 on the pH scale and is generally considered acidic.

5) Whole-body immersion therapy: A recent study in the Journal of Experimental Medicine looked at this treatment and found it very effective. It helped increase muscle mass and improve bone density.

6) Fasting: During a fast diet, you are forced to eat as little as necessary to keep your body alive for your body's natural ability to start breaking down fat stores for energy. This causes your body's pH levels to naturally lower, making it easier for your body to shed weight or gain muscle.

Note that these treatments cannot be done in isolation. They must work in conjunction with one another to ensure you receive the proper amount of nutrients and minerals your body needs to maintain a healthy, alkaline pH balance.

Chapter 11:

Alkaline Plant Foods and Herbs Support

I f you want to live a healthier life, we recommend adopting a diet rich in alkaline foods and herbs. Alkalinity is the opposite of acidity, and the body has specific mechanisms for regulating blood pH. When these systems are working correctly, there is little or no impact on health. If these systems break down as they can do with aging or illness, acidosis can develop. Acidosis is linked to many health problems, including anxiety, depression, insomnia, and other sleep disorders.

The Alkaline Diet not only promotes optimal health but also helps prevent illness and disease. Alkaline foods and herbs support the immune system by providing more oxygen for cells to metabolize toxins and produce life-sustaining energy.

Although it's easy to get confused by all the different terms and recommendations, a healthy alkaline diet is not hard to adopt. As well as its many proven health benefits, the benefits of eating and drinking alkaline foods are just as practical for helping to lose weight. The average body pH is slightly alkaline at about 7.4–7.6, and the ideal body pH range is between 7.8 and 8.5.

Alkalinity refers to a substance's ability to neutralize the acid in the body or raise overall pH levels when ingested. The food you eat can impact your blood's pH levels because your blood must maintain a certain level of acidity for optimum health: this level resides somewhere between 7.36 and 7.45. This threshold pH is often referred to as the "ideal" or baseline blood pH. When blood pH levels fall below 7.35, it is called acidosis, and when it rises above 7.45, it is called alkalosis.

What Are Alkaline Foods and Herbs?

Alkaline-forming foods are naturally rich in minerals and help balance our bodies' pH and are alkalizing. Foods that increase the acidity in our bodies are called acid-forming foods, including meat, sugar, grains, dairy products, and other processed foods. Even though fruits contain natural sugar, their high levels of antioxidants make them excellent for balancing blood pH levels.

Alkaline-forming herbs have a differentiating effect on the body. More than 80 alkalizing herbs have been used for thousands of years for one or more of their many health benefits. The alkaloids in these plants help restore the body's pH balance, and they are very effective in preventing many health problems.

We're here to tell you about alkaline plant foods and how they support health. Acidic diets have been shown to increase acid levels in the body, leading to adverse health consequences such as weight gain and osteoporosis. Many people believe the Alkaline Diet is the way of restoring balance by reducing acidity in the body. To achieve this balance, alkaline plants act as a buffer and help neutralize any acidic effects from other foods you might eat. In general, it's essential for everyone - not just those who struggle with health issues related to being too acidic - to know about these alkaline plant foods so they can maintain an optimal level of pH in their bodies.

pH is a scientific measurement that describes the acidity or alkalinity of a solution. Solutions with lower pH values are acidic, while those with higher values are said to be alkaline. Why is this important? Even mild acidity has been linked to infertility and respiratory problems, and severe bites can lead to death. Certain disease states can be brought on by too much acidity in the body, resulting in one or more symptoms being caused by having too much acid in the blood. This is usually referred to as 'metabolic acidosis.

Are there certain alkaline foods?

Many types of food are alkaline. Using a scale of 1-14, where seven is neutral, and anything below is acidic, raw fruits and vegetables generally fall between 7 and 10, with some exceptions. Some examples of these alkaline foods include:

• Apples

• Limes

• Carrots

• Parsley

Some plant foods aren't as high on the pH scale. These foods are more acidic in studies. Some examples of these foods are:

• Tomatoes

- Bell Peppers

- Cucumbers

- Celery

What are some alkaline herbs? Not all plant foods are fruits and vegetables. Herbs, like plants, also fall on a scale of 1-14, where seven is neutral. The scale is slightly different for condiments because some are much more alkaline than others. The general rule with herbs is that they should be used in moderation. That's because any herbs you use will affect your body's pH level, and if they're too high, they can potentially cause issues in the long term.

Some of the highest alkaline herbal teas are:

- Hibiscus flower

- Nettle root

- Rosehips

- Dandelion root

Of course, too much of anything can be harmful. Not necessarily! You just have to use moderation to avoid potential problems. You should always use your common sense and be careful around anything you're introduced to for the first time. Too much of anything might lead to any of the following: dizziness/unsteadiness, nausea, diarrhea, stomachache or headache, unusual tiredness or fatigue, heavy sweating or thirst, vomiting, and elevated heartbeat.

Importance of Alkaline Plant Foods and Herbs Support

Why is it that alkaline plant food and herbal support are so important? The answer lies in the make-up of our blood. Our blood pH should ideally be around 7.35; this is slightly alkaline, which gives us all the nutrition we need to function correctly, whether we're tired or not. When our body gets acidic, though, eventually, we'll find ourselves struggling with various ailments. All unhealthy foods are acidic, meat being one of the worst, for example. The more acidity in our body, the worse it becomes as time goes by, and eventually, health problems will develop if nothing changes.

We just can't have a plant food-only diet. When we eat more acid-forming foods like meats, grains, dairy products, etc., our food takes far to digest. This causes us to feel heavier and very "full" after eating smaller portions during meals, which will slow down our metabolism levels and increase stress hormones such as cortisol, which inhibits thyroid hormone action in the body.

As we get older, the metabolites from eating acid-forming foods can become toxic to the body and stimulate disease. Also, as we age, our ability to use enzymes will decrease, which means that our bodies will take longer to digest protein, for example.

Many people are still eating a diet of main meat, flour-based carbohydrate foods, and poor quality vegetable oils which are low in essential fatty acids and vitamins, to name but a few. They put on weight quickly, their immune systems become less effective, and they suffer from the degenerative diseases of aging. Their metabolism is slowed down, leaving them feeling tired and generally unwell.

Alkaline plant foods and herbs help to help the body achieve and maintain a natural state of balance. This balance is essential for our overall health because the body can resist disease during times of stress and illness when it has an alkaline environment. On the other hand, an alkaline environment in your body will help your cells to absorb oxygen more effectively, and cell membranes will remain tighter, so they take up less space.

A diet high in alkaline foods and herbs promotes good health because it improves the ability of the body to maintain a healthy pH level naturally. This helps to prevent acid-forming chemicals from getting into our bodies which can cause neurotoxicity or damage. A healthy pH level is also essential for our mental well-being, mood, and clear thinking too.

A healthy alkaline state can help:

1. Reduce fatigue and increase energy

2. Improve digestion and bowel function

3. Maintain healthy skin and hair

4. Improve mood and reduce depression and anxiety

The human body is an ecosystem, and the types of food we eat will affect its balance. To keep our bodies in balance, we need to consume an alkaline-forming diet. Put into perspective, an apple would have a pH of 3.5 while a potato would measure at 4.0 on the same scale, both considered as "acidic.

The acidic foods we eat have a significant influence on the pH of body tissue; acidity causes disease. We require an alkaline pH of at least 7.365 to be healthy and maintain good health. If our diet is too acidic, it causes a drop in blood pH, resulting in a less than optimal function of enzymes and other body components. An acidic environment also encourages the growth of harmful microbes (disease). Ensuring that our daily nutritional intake is alkaline-forming helps ensure that our bodies function at their highest level to enjoy good health for more extended periods. What we eat will determine if our blood pH levels are acidic or alkaline.

Each day our bodies fight the effects of stress, pollution, and other environmental toxins. In doing so, it becomes depleted of essential minerals, vitamins, and nutrients. These biochemical building blocks that help the body repair damaged tissue and maintain proper health in a highly acidic environment become less available when the body is under stress. Research has shown that our dietary intake of acid buffering minerals such as calcium, magnesium, and potassium declines significantly as we age. The alkalizing minerals that help neutralize the acidity of foods are what we should be eating more to maintain a healthy body pH balance.

Alkalizing plant foods include:

Green vegetables and sprouts, which can be eaten raw, steamed, or sautéed. Carrot juice is also a portion of good alkalinizing food as it naturally has a pH of 8.0 or higher because of its high sugar content and the high sodium content of carrots (salt has a pH of 9.0). The degree to which an item is alkaline-forming can be determined by looking at its pH value against the diet acid balance scale. This means that green leafy vegetables such as kale have a higher alkalizing potential than root vegetables such as carrots or potatoes. Equally important is the optimization of the ratio of potassium to sodium in our diet.

Chlorophyll is the primary substance in green leafy vegetables that creates an alkalizing effect. It is a green pigment found in chlorophyll-containing plants, and it helps keep the body's pH neutral. Chlorophyll protects against oxidative damage to cells, making it a valuable ally in the fight against aging and disease.

Legumes are high in proteins and complex carbohydrates that help to keep blood sugar levels steady after eating. Beans also contain potassium, which acts as an alkalizing mineral.

Nuts and seeds, which are concentrated alkaline foods, contain many essential minerals. Because they focus on alkaline foods, it is necessary not to overconsume them or go overboard eating large amounts of nuts and seeds regularly.

Drinking an ounce of lemon juice in water first thing in the morning is an excellent alkalizing practice that will reduce acidosis.

Chapter 12:

How to Detox Using Alkaline Foods and pH Balance Diet

Y ou look great, but you still feel awful, sluggish, and foggy. It's time to detox! You may be wondering how to detox or what the benefits of detoxing are. Detoxing is a natural process your body does to clean out any potentially toxic substances that could inhibit your organs from performing correctly.

Detoxifying can include removing unwanted chemicals, candida, surface metals accumulated from eating acidic foods that keep the body in an inflammatory state, and other forms of waste, including fecal matter stored in the colon. Detoxification is how cells can get rid of waste materials that may have built up in their system. We were told that you needed to consume more acidic foods to detoxify for years, but this is not true!

The human body is a complicated system, and it's difficult to imagine how any single food can be excellent or horrible for it. But that doesn't mean that some foods don't have more of an advantage than others. Some people, however, think that returning the pH level in the body back to natural alkaline levels will help decrease inflammation. And while this does seem like something worth investigating because of all the benefits that alkaline foods offer, like helping your digestion and providing powerful antioxidants for your immune system, there is no research backing up any specific diet as a "detox food."

The Alkaline Diet is the most popular detox diet. Alkaline foods are said to have a much more beneficial effect on the body than acidic foods. In many cases, a powerful Alkaline Diet will help improve various health conditions and bring your body back into balance. You have learned what foods are best for detoxing and how certain types can increase your energy levels as well as your physical health.

Why should I be detoxing, and how does it help me? After all, we are told that the body "cleans itself" naturally as our metabolism, water, and other fluids naturally flush toxins through our body. The problem with this is that we have toxins in our bodies that are not being removed! Think about it. Have you ever had a drink and then felt like you were poisoned? This is the result of toxins in your system not being cleared. The toxins stay trapped inside your body, hurting you no matter how much water, exercise, or fruit you drink.

Are you dreaming about how great it will be to increase weight loss through detoxing? Well, first of all, we don't need to lose weight! Detoxing helps us get rid of waste and toxic materials.

It's essential to have a healthy lifestyle. When you have an average pH level and a healthy diet, you feel good and look vibrant with shiny hair and glowing skin - not to mention all the energy you have!

When you adjust your pH to a healthier level, you experience a lasting quality of life. The Alkaline Diet can help repair areas in the body that have become damaged by oxidative stress or unhealthy nutrition. This is because body cells can repair themselves when the body is in balance and receive adequate nutrition. The main reason the Alkaline Diet is so effective is that it returns to your body's natural pH, somewhere around 7.35-7.45, which has been proven by science to be what your body can repair itself into naturally when there are no outside influences on its pH.

The pH diet: What you can eat

Before changing your diet, it is recommended that you check your pH balance with a saliva test kit or urinalysis - these can be purchased at any drugstore. When doing a saliva test, you need to have freshly drawn saliva because the saliva pH levels will change during the day and after eating. After you get a read on your pH, you can begin making changes.

The ideal food choices are those that are alkaline-forming. A food with a pH of 8 or higher is considered alkaline-forming, and those under pH 7 are acid-forming. You can eat plenty of fresh fruits and vegetables, whole grains, legumes, nuts, and seeds to your heart's content! However, meats are more challenging to digest, making them harder for the body to break down into smaller particles to be absorbed into the cells. Dairy products such as milk, cheese, and yogurt should also be avoided since they are considered acid-forming. However, yogurt is a better option than regular milk since it has probiotics that help restore your gut health.

Alkaline-forming foods include:

Vegetables: all leafy greens, like spinach and kale; broccoli; cauliflower; celery; cabbage; cucumber.

Fruits: berries such as blueberries and blackberries are very alkaline-forming; peaches, mangos, apples, and pears are also excellent choices. Berries such as blueberries and blackberries are very alkaline-forming; peaches, mangos, apples, and pears are also excellent choices.

Grains: quinoa and amaranth are alkaline-forming grains that you can eat in moderation. Other grains, like wheat and corn, are acid-forming, so they should be eaten only in moderation or not at all.

Quinoa and amaranth are alkaline-forming grains that you can eat in moderation. Other grains, like wheat and corn, are acid-forming, so they should be eaten only in moderation or not at all. Legumes: all legumes, except for soybeans, are alkaline forming.

All legumes, except for soybeans, are alkaline forming. Nuts and seeds: almonds; peanuts; walnuts; sunflower seeds.

Herbs and spices contain a multitude of healing properties and are very alkaline forming. Some examples include garlic, ginger root, cilantro, black pepper, and turmeric that have anti-inflammatory effects on the body!

Dairy products: milk, yogurt, and cheese should be avoided; instead, drink a glass of unsweetened almond milk to get the calcium you need.

Milk, yogurt, and cheese should be avoided; instead, drink a glass of unsweetened almond milk to get the calcium you need.

Like any other non-vegetarian food, alcohol should be limited to no more than two drinks per day. As with any other non-vegetarian food, alcohol should be limited to no more than two drinks per day.

Sugary foods: anything high in sugar should be avoided. This includes all processed foods and overly sweetened fruit juices. Instead, focus on eating whole fruits and vegetables. These will help to alkalize your body, but they are also a great source of vitamins, minerals, and fiber, which helps keep insulin levels low, which helps with weight loss!

Alkaline-forming foods can balance the body's pH levels by alkalizing the body, while acid-forming foods will acidify it. The ideal pH ranges for adults are between 6 and 7; this is what you want to aim for! To check your pH levels or some other considerations when it comes to diet, visit www.naturalhealthybodyguide.com.

Your body is comprised of numerous components, and all must work together for you to live healthily at an optimal level. The digestive system, nervous system, and endocrine system - along with the liver and gallbladder - all work together daily to create a healthy life every day.

As is the case with most things, if your system is not working correctly, it won't be too long before we begin to feel sick and start having health issues. As a result, we need to balance our body's internal pH regularly to remain efficient at all times. Once we get out of balance, we need to know how to get back to the correct pH to feel better. This is why it is so important to get yourself into an alkaline state regularly. This is something that can be done in the comfort of your own home or with the help of a professional.

Are you acidified? The balance between alkalinity and acidity needs to be maintained for optimum health, which begins by understanding its pH balance. In addition to dieting for better food selection, a whole-body approach includes healthy habits such as meditation or yoga – or any other way of managing stress levels. It's also essential to maintain proper hydration levels. Water is the key to alkalinity, and drinking enough water allows the body to function at its best.

We lose a lot of our water every day through breathing, sweating, and elimination through urination. If you have inadequate hydration, this can lead to acidity – a type of derangement that is very common in America today! The pH scale uses 0 to 14 to measure the acidity or alkalinity of substances. Normal pH levels range from 1-6; anything below 7 (acidic) or above 7 (alkaline) is considered unhealthy. Sugar and carbohydrates are both very sour, so a diet rich in these types of foods can lead to acidity.

How to detox with alkaline foods and pH balanced diet.

You can address acidity anywhere in your body with many different techniques, but there are two that stand out: alkaline foods and pH balanced diet. Both have been used as a natural way of detoxing for centuries. The alkaline food technique is the best way to begin the process of rebalancing the body's pH balance since it includes plenty of alkaline vegetables and fruits grown at higher pH levels. Alkaline foods are grown in greenhouses, which are kept at a higher pH level. They often include apple juice, molasses, and Rumney Creek Mangosteen juice. These fresh alkaline foods work best against acidity, especially if you're not eating enough protein.

It's best to start with an organic diet that doesn't contain sugar and processed carbohydrates. Remember to drink two big glasses of pure water every day – one at mealtime and the other before bedtime for best results!

Differences Between an Alkaline Diet and Ph Balanced Diet

One of the main differences between the Alkaline Diet and a pH-balanced diet is that the former focuses on a minimal number of foods, while the latter offers lots of fresh fruits and vegetables to eat. The Alkaline Diet (permaculture) emphasizes natural cultivation methods such as permaculture, aquaculture, mushroom growing, etc. This integrates the practices of healthy food cultivation into a lifestyle that avoids toxins in food and water.

The pH-balanced diet has taken the best aspects of the Alkaline Diet and added more natural whole foods with higher pH levels (pH 11- 12). Alkaline foods range from whole grain cereals to dark chocolate and even fruits and vegetables. This is a beautiful way to detox since it allows the body to eliminate toxins through the kidneys and bowels, organs that cannot do so.

Chapter 13:

How to Fight Diseases Using Alkaline Foods and a pH Balanced Diet

D id you know that what you eat has a significant effect on health and wellness? One of the most effective ways to improve your health is by including foods with an alkaline pH balance in your diet. Eat right to stay healthy. This is true, but not enough people realize that there are many different ways in which the foods they eat can affect their health. The most common example is acid-forming food versus alkaline-forming food and its effect on the body's pH balance.

Alkaline foods refer to a diet that emphasizes vegetables, fruits, and other plant-based foods with an alkaline pH of 7 or higher. This dietary system has gained popularity due to its alleged benefits in the fight against diseases like cancer. The theory behind the Alkaline Diet is that by eating food with a high pH, you can restore your body's natural acid/alkaline balance, which is essential for good health. The idea is based on research done nearly 100 years ago by Nobel Prize winner Otto Warburg who noticed that most cancer cells thrive in an acidic environment.

The Alkaline Diet is supposed to improve health by increasing antioxidant levels and reducing inflammation. It has been linked to weight loss and an increase in longevity since a high pH allows your body to extract more nutrients from food. The findings suggest that it's possible to eat a high-pH diet (which is also low in animal fats) to reverse aging and fighting diseases like cancer.

The Alkaline Diet is an excellent alternative to other diets like the Paleo diet rich in protein, but it is lacking in many essential vitamins and minerals. Plus, the high-fat content of the paleo diet could lead to osteoporosis later on. The body's pH balance plays a significant role in almost all diseases. The well-balanced Alkaline Diet will help keep your pH balanced and prevent diseases such as heart disease, diabetes, hypertension, osteoporosis, arthritis, and cancer.

You can safely produce alkaline ash in your body by taking wheatgrass juices, drinking water infused with lemon and lime juice, and eating alkalizing fruits and vegetables. "Alkaline ash" are the alkaline salts formed when you break down simple sugars and complex carbohydrates containing mainly fructose, galactose, glucose, and maltose. These sugars have an abundance of acidic hydrogen ions. When we break down these sugars (ex. refined sugar), the formation of these alkaline salts is what regulates our pH balance. The disruption of this natural process, which produces alkaline salts as a byproduct, can lead to acidosis, which is common in our day and age.

The Alkaline Diet is so helpful in keeping your body's pH balanced because every single cellular system in your body, including those vital for the proper functioning of your brain and nervous system, requires an alkaline pH range. For example, a healthy cell membrane must be acidic to allow the cell's internal machinery to function correctly.

An acidic quality or pH level of 7 or below is associated with heart disease. Simultaneously, highly alkalizing foods help maintain an alkaline pH within the tissues of our bodies and organs. An acidic quality or pH level of 7 or below is associated with heart disease. Simultaneously, highly alkalizing foods help maintain an alkaline pH within the tissues of our bodies and organs.

Where do we get the necessary building blocks for an alkaline-forming diet? Almost all of these foods are readily available on nearly any grocery store's shelves, so you should not find it challenging to incorporate these into your busy lifestyle.

Some of the best sources for an Alkaline Diet include grains, beans, nuts, seeds, fruits, and vegetables. You can buy wheatgrass juice in most health food stores. There are many brands out there, and they may vary in quality and price. I'd recommend buying it from a health food store rather than the grocery store, as you are more likely to find better quality wheatgrass there. You can find quality juice that is not made with heat or pressure pasteurization and is very fresh. Chlorella is also a portion of great alkalizing food. It has been shown to reduce free radical damage, and it's an excellent source of protein and chlorophyll.

Limiting acidic or inflammatory foods is also suitable for balancing your pH levels. Highly acidic or inflammatory foods should be limited in the diet or avoided altogether. Here is some information on how to reduce your intake of inflammatory foods:

Alcoholic beverages: Beer can be as acidic as vinegar, depending on the ingredients used in making it. Certain alcoholic beverages may cause acidosis and increase the body's acid load. Alcohol also contributes to dehydration and is a direct toxin to our bodies.

Artificial sweeteners, sugar and processed foods tend to increase acid levels in the body more than possible alkalizing foods would, so they should be avoided altogether.

Caffeine or caffeine-containing goods (coffee, tea, chocolate). Caffeine is one of the most harmful foods you can eat. Caffeine causes increased cell death and liver damage. It reduces antioxidant levels, making it even more important to avoid caffeine (both coffee and natural stimulants) if you are looking to detoxify your body and remove existing toxins. Caffeine increases cortisol, which is a chemical stress hormone that contributes to accelerated aging. Theobromine, an ingredient in chocolate similar to caffeine but acts more slowly in the body, can increase heart rate and blood pressure.

Alcoholic beverages are also part of this category as they cause dehydration in your body and contain sugar, which can feed yeast infections or candida issues, further contributing to inflammation.

Artificial sweeteners have been shown to increase obesity, Type 2 diabetes, and heart disease when used in place of natural sugar. Aspartame has been linked to cancer (as have many other artificial sweeteners). Artificially sweetened foods and drinks are now being studied to contribute to diseases such as lupus, multiple sclerosis, memory loss, and concentration problems.

Foods containing preservatives or additives:

Many processed foods contain additives that increase the acidity within your body. For example, many lunch meats contain nitrites (an additive preservative), while some cheeses contain a common food additive called cellulose powder which is also very acidic.

Here is a list of common food additives and preservatives you should avoid:

Sulfites keep dried fruits, frozen dinners, nuts, seeds, and dehydrated potato products fresh for more extended periods.

Carrageenan is used as an emulsifier in many ice creams. It comes from seaweed which has been treated with extremely high heat and pressure. Carrageenan is a toxin that can stimulate immune reactions even at low ingestion levels (in the range of 1-100 ng/g).

Cyclamate is a sweetener used in many processed foods and drinks. It may cause headaches, abdominal cramps, and nervousness and interfere with regular insulin and thyroid function.

These additives are used to preserve the food from spoilage or decomposition. Unfortunately, these preservatives can produce free radicals, which increase the body's acidic state. Some of the more common ingredients used in preserving food include:

Acids or acid-forming foods:

The foods listed below contain high levels of natural acid-forming substances that contribute to an acidic system in your body, which is not suitable for you.

Grapes, raisins, and wine are good examples of acidic foods. Unlike most other fruits, they are made up of the sugar fructose, easily converted by the body into a chemical called uric acid. Uric acid is found in your joints, and when it accumulates in significant quantities, it can lead to gout.

Other acidic foods:

Sugar (white sugar), oligofructoses - especially short-chain oligofructoses such as maltose and sucrose - and lactose.

Certain types of fruit - namely apples, pears, peaches, and strawberries - contain important estrogen hormones. These hormones can disrupt your body's natural processes if eaten in large quantities.

Beans and legumes. Even though they are a great source of plant protein and fiber are also very high in phytic acid, which inhibits the absorption of minerals such as iron, zinc, calcium, and magnesium.

Fermented foods such as sauerkraut and other vegetable ferments contain foodborne microorganisms that can contribute to indigestion and digestive problems.

Foods that suppress the immune function:

The leading cause of an acidic condition in our bodies is a disruption in the body's pH balance. The disruption of this natural process can lead to a condition called acidosis. Three primary factors are contributing to the trouble of this balance:

A loss of dietary alkaline-forming foods in combination with an excess of acidic forming foods. Consumption of mineral or vitamin supplements without enough food energy, leading to a shortage of pH-sustaining minerals or vitamins in the system. Consumption of excessive amounts of caffeine.

Suppressing your immune function makes it easy for pathogens such as bacteria, viruses, and parasites to disrupt your body's normal biological processes and cause disease. When the immune system is suppressed, your cells are continuously exposed to dangerous pathogens, leading to immune dysfunction and disease.

The most common cause of an acidic pH in the body is excessive consumption of acidic foods, mainly processed foods. An acidic pH has also been linked to a more generally unhealthy lifestyle, including a diet high in sugar and fat, inadequate physical activity, and excessive alcohol consumption. These lifestyle choices contribute to acidosis by creating an environment that is not conducive to the intestine and pancreas' optimal function.

Don't overeat acidic food because it causes your body to use extra energy to keep its pH balance.

How you can change this by eating more alkaline foods. This is basically what Dr. Robert Young had figured out when he created his pH-balanced diet system. His book "The pH Miracle for Weight Loss" is all about how he's used alkaline foods as an aid for losing weight. He also wrote The pH Miracle, geared toward expanding human potential through diet and lifestyle choices.

The Mediterranean Diet is another way to eat more alkaline foods. A diet that includes fish, yogurt, feta cheese, whole grains, and vegetables.

Let's talk about what your body does if you don't eat acid-forming foods. When we don't eat enough alkaline foods, our bodies go into a state of shock. Our metabolism slows down because our cells stop taking up glucose (sugar), converting them into ketones instead. Ketones are the primary fuel for our brains and organs, and anything that doesn't store glucose in the body goes into ketogenesis.

The benefits of the Alkaline Diet are not just limited to the prevention of disease. Other benefits include:

-Increased energy levels by having more oxygen in the blood

-Better digestion by producing more hydrochloric acid in our stomachs

-Better elimination of toxins by digesting protein more efficiently

-Fewer muscle cramps when exercising by having more calcium in the body

-Better breathing and better quality sleep. We breathe alkalized air during the day, and when we sleep, we can improve our breathing at night.

If one is eating many alkaline foods and taking many supplements, it is unnecessary or desirable to take extra calcium to prevent bone loss. Calcium will build up in the body if there aren't enough alkaline minerals in the diet to absorb it.

Conclusion

A lkaline dieting is a way to detoxify and fight disease by eating alkaline foods. The diet's purpose is keeping our body at a pH balance ideal for healing, and it entails consuming different alkaline substances to neutralize acidity, mostly caused by consumption of animal products, refined sugars, and processed foods. Veganism helps with this issue because plant-based food alone does not produce any acidity in the stomach. Therefore, alkalizing the diet from protein to plant-based food is a great way to heal the body from chronic disease.

The principles of the Alkaline Diet are simple: eating real foods with a pH level close to 10 or above. This means we want to eat fruits, vegetables, nuts and seeds, and legumes to achieve balance. The purpose of the diet is to improve health by making our body alkaline and avoid illness because these foods are loaded with nutrients that prevent disease and create a strong body.

We are what we eat. This statement is true in every sense of the word. Our body is made up of the food we consume, and if it is not helpful to our health, it will have a negative impact on our future. Yet, most of us do not even consider this when eating meals or consuming snacks. People need to learn to control themselves from eating junk food created by big corporations just so they can make more money off all of us with poor health.

It is possible to maintain a lifestyle where you get enough nutrients while still eating delicious foods every day to prevent any disease from developing in your body. You can avoid chronic disease by eating the right foods and beverages that alkalize the body. The foundation of a healthy eating routine is to eliminate acid-producing foods, such as meat, dairy, baked goods, soda, coffee and alcohol while balancing meals with alkaline-producing fruits and vegetables.

This does not mean you have to deny yourself anything you love; it simply means you must choose the right kind of food. Each day we are faced with choices as to what we will put in our body, and for many it is hard to distinguish between what is good for our health or bad for us.

Following the Alkaline Diet is great way to achieve long-lasting health. The best way is by educating yourself on what foods are good for your body and what to avoid. Just like everything else, there is a right and a wrong answer. We all have different bodies that react differently to things, but the core principles of the Alkaline Diet can be practiced by almost everyone no matter who you are.

It only matters that you are willing to take the initiative to change your lifestyle to achieve better health and live longer. If you are looking to improve the overall quality of your health, I highly recommend you look into Alkaline Dieting as a way to accomplish this goal. It can seem overwhelming in the beginning or even confusing, but if you take it one step at a time, you will reach your final goal. This is not a diet that promotes quick results; it takes time to see any significant changes in your health because it is about changing your eating habits for the long run.

Last, but not least, know that any change is hard but worth it. If you are really serious about being healthier, then switching over to the Alkaline Diet is something you should strongly consider.

Remember that no matter what, it only matters that you are willing to make a change.

CPSIA information can be obtained
at www.ICGtesting.com
Printed in the USA
LVHW080814030622
720418LV00008B/323